"Explores the relationship between the foods we consume and the way we feel."

– Matthew Kenney, author of *Cooked Raw*

Nourished

The Plant-based Path to Health & Happiness

Pamela Wasabi

Preface by Matthew Kenney, author of *Cooked Raw*

Para Margarita
La más sabia de las flores.
Ella, quien ha visto el crecer, llorar, y el amar
y la metamorfosis de cuatro generaciones.

Te adoro.

"Nourished is one of those books that feels HOME the moment that you pick it up. Visually and verbally it acknowledges and inspires the creator in all of us to commune deeply with life via the food we consume and the way we consume it."

- Jenna Johnson,
Embodiment Coach and
Creator of LooksGoodOnYouInc

"Pamela not only has an enormous knowledge of plant based cuisine, she is also an amazing cook and shares a message that goes with every dish. The message of self-love, self-nourishing, self-awareness towards a better and conscious way of eating. Only through our own self love and awareness we will heal ourselves, I trust Pamela for every dish to show me the amazing power that food have in our physical bodies and souls."

- Mariana Cortez,
Founder and Owner of Bunnie Cakes

"You are the sum total of everything you've ever seen, heard, eaten, smelled, been told, forgot – it's all there. Everything influences each of us, and because of that I try to make sure that my experiences are positive."

-Maya Angelou

Table of Contents

Preface   11

Foreword   13

Introduction   15

Dirt
                                           16
    Milk   19
    Salsa de Tomate   21
    [Burnt] Mushroom Soup   24
    Chicken Nugget   26
    Cold Turkey   28
    Eggs and Bacon   29
    Tofu   31

Seed
                                           34
    Carob   37
    Decaf Coffee   39
    Love   40
    Hungry   41
    Fear   42
    Sunfoods   43
    Faith   45
    Relaxation   46
    Maca   47
    Breastmilk   49
    Violetta   50

Root
                                           52
    Coconut Water   55
    Placenta Pills   57
    Chocolate Oat Cookie   58
    Gut   59

Mango Custard   60
Gluten-Free   62
Umami   64
Sugar   66
Meatless Monday   69
Chef   71

Sprout   74
Kale   77
Plate   80
Sun   83
Blood   87
Harmony   91
Honey   94
Kraut   97
Seasons   100

Fruit   106
Chopsticks   109
Kitchen   111
Relationship with Food   113

Bloom   114
Nourished   117
#Nourishedpath   119
Nourished Tips   120

Conclusion   121

Plant-Based Recipes   123

Acknowledgments   173

Author Bio   175

Nourished

Preface

"Congratulations to Pamela on launching *Nourished*, It is always an honor to connect with similar pioneers in the plant-based community and I am especially proud of our alumni who are doing wonderful work to improve global health. *Nourished* explores the relationship between the foods we consume and the way we feel. This concept was instrumental in my transition to a fully plant-based diet and lifestyle. These topics inspire and challenge readers to become more conscious about their choices and ultimately support our main goal of reducing animal consumption around the world."

– Matthew Kenney,
Plant Based Celebrity Chef, Author

Nourished

Foreword

My personal journey into holistic living began 11 years ago with an E3 live blue-green algae shot and a yoga instructor named Fred Busch on Miami Beach. From that day forward, my life was headed down a new path. Living consciously and holistically has changed my life in every single facet—literally. Most of my life I struggled with obesity and diabetes and was living a completely different lifestyle with a mindset quite different than the one from today. It was not until I adopted this new lifestyle, incorporating many modalities of health and healing, that I truly found happiness and comfort in my own mind body and spirit.

The change – an evolution – was on a cellular level. After experiencing this in my own life, I knew in my heart I needed to bring it to others by offering our community a center for holistic transformation. This is why I created The Sacred Space Miami.

The Sacred Space is an oasis in the heart of the city of Miami offering many modalities of healing and education. Our campus includes Plant Food + Wine and Matthew Kenney Culinary; the city's first and only classically structured plant-based culinary academy. The restaurant and culinary institute are an integral part of The Sacred Space Miami, aligning perfectly with the larger mission: combining health, education and community.

Whether having a plant-based meal with friends at Plant Food + Wine, or attending a Shamanic Journey or transformational workshop, The Sacred Space is truly a center for integrated experiences. Furthermore, the space is a reflection of my personal belief system and the holistic way in which I live my life.

This mindset of a holistic life is tied to being a mindful person. Mindfulness is vigilant awareness of being in the present moment. So often we live in the past and future and that can be terribly dangerous. Ask yourself this, do you know what exists there? What do you imagine lives in the past and in the present? For many, it is suffering.

Being aware is living in the moment, and that's the only place that exists. It's really about savoring the present moment—the Now.

And that's where Pamela comes in. Pamela is one of the most mindful and present human beings I have ever come across. I met Pamela when she came to support the Plant Food + Wine culinary team during the South Beach Food and Wine Festival dinner at The Sacred Space. The moment I met her I sensed her passion, deep understanding and enthusiasm around her craft.

She worked with *Jugo*Fresh R&D kitchen pop-up, and was involved with the pioneers in the conscious and plant-based scene in the city. Pamela now actively teaches workshops at The Sacred Space Miami and also has led a Conscious Bite Out dinner in our space.

Not only was I hearing about her belief system and the fabulous work she was doing—I witnessed and experienced it firsthand. We were continuously seeing each other through our shared passion for holistic living, and our relationship evolved into one where I entrusted her expertise and sought out her advice explicitly as my in-house chef.

I had such faith in Pamela from the moment we started working together, and she—along with her beautiful "helper" daughter, Violetta—began delivering weekly meals for my family. The best part about having Pamela's food delivered daily (asides from the convenience) was knowing every aspect was holistically prepared, and all ingredients were plant-based and healthy. People often think plant-based food means lacks flavor or some part of the experience is sacrificed. Pamela continuously impressed me with the crafting of unbelievably complex and satiating plant-based food to the point I would call some dishes comfort food!

On top of that, everything was created with a lot of integrity and blessings—I could sense the love and commitment put into every dish, with every bite. That love behind her skills are only the beginning. As you'll see as you turn the page, Pamela is more than a chef. She's a mother, giver and a teacher. She is not only passionate about her craft, she is passion. The way she treats her body and nourishes it, should be an example for us all. She believes in her philosophies and lives her life in alignment. Not only is she naturally attuned towards holistic living, she is also so well educated and possesses the credentials to back it. Her knowledge transcends beyond being a plant-based chef, and delves into areas of holistic nutrition and the psychology of eating. It's incredibly inspiring seeing how she lives her life with such integrity, balance and harmony with plant-based living and nature.

Karla Dascal is the founder of The Sacred Space Miami, an epicenter for personal growth and transformation in the dynamic Wynwood Arts District. The Sacred Space is home to plant-based eatery Plant Food + Wine Miami, and the raw living food academy, Matthew Kenney Culinary.

Introduction

"This book is a guide and example of change. *Nourished* is about the journey and responsibility we have to our bodies, our happiness, and our planet. It invites us to listen closely to our relationship with food, to rescue our family and cultural values through cooking, and to understand that we are all part of Nature. *Nourished* is living in harmony with food, health and the Earth."

This idea appreciates the diversity of our planet, our different cultures and our heritage. I don't want to instill dogmatic thinking in you. I just hope that together we can analyze any school of thought from a distance and take from it the underlying principle of its wisdom. Being plant-based myself, the meaning of my lifestyle and what I intend to spread with this book is awareness, love and gratitude.

For 10 years or so I dealt with a thyroid imbalance, which I now recognize as a catalyst for change. When I finally decided to educate myself and handle health as my responsibility, my life took a turn to healing, plant based cooking, and sharing valuable information and expanding the minds of those I encounter on my path.

I've organized this book to mimic the growth of a plant and to resemble the phases I went through in moving towards my own evolution. Subdividing these stages into subchapters, I named each segment after the food or feeling that symbolized my "hunger" at the time.

The growth stages of a plant demonstrate the phases that all living beings go through as change happens, including Nature. Probably the most valuable underlying lesson we can learn from Mother Earth is to admit that no matter who or where in life we are, change is constant, and so is our never-ending growth and improvement.

Throughout the chapters I have scattered basic plant-based recipes and cooking techniques to help you defeat your fear in the kitchen, fear that I overcame when I understood that cooking is therapy and that cooking is the best thing you can do for your health.

To your Nourished Path,
Pamela Wasabi

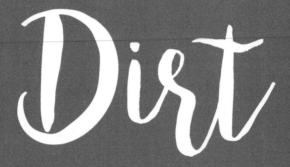

"For a seed to achieve its greatest expression it must come completely undone. The shell cracks. Its insides come out and everything changes. To someone who doesn't understand growth, it would look like complete destructions."

— Cynthia Occelli

milk

You are what you eat, they say. How far are we willing to take that statement? Let's face it, food is what makes the world turn – not money. We actually work to "bring home the bacon" or to "put bread on the table". Every minute that goes by we are digesting food, converting food into usable energy, or longing for the next meal. Our family celebrations and our national holidays are all around dinner tables and cookouts. We eat to survive, but we may also eat for nourishment, and we can also eat for punishment, or to fill a void.

Food has different meanings for each one of us. We all have a relationship with food that is distinctly individual and complex. For some, food may be a symbol of love and pleasure. It can be something positive or negative. Food may simply be fuel. Food provides energy. It can bring life or death. For me, from my earliest memories on my journey to this moment as I type these words, food has meant a search for belonging, finding home.

I still remember sucking on my mother's breast. She was my home. My mom provided me much more than just food with her milk then; I tasted her nurturing heart and warmth, which kept me on her lap and in her arms till I was 4. Soon after, I transitioned to cow's milk, my eye-opener and daily breakfast before school. I associated milk with health, with doing the right thing. Whatever that meant to me at that young age, the responsibility of taking care of my body was already instilled in me, a value that has accompanied me and helped me transform myself from sickness and sadness to making a career around nourishing the world.

Milk is associated with feminine energy, in Ayurvedic medicine, dairy is part of the Ayurveda vegetarian diet because it provides a nourishing and calming energy. Milk is such a precious and sacred drink, it represents "progress". It's derived from the mother, the creator and main provider for a young child's growth and development. It's the most natural form of food to help a kid "progress" from the first instant after emerging from the womb to the baby's first cognitive moments. It's a complete food that comes with all of the essential nutrients that a baby needs while at mother's breast. The connection of the baby's saliva to the mom's nipple communicates exactly what the baby needs so that the mother's system can adapt, create, and specifically provide. There's so much beauty in breast-feeding. It is Nature interacting with us, elongating the course of our evolution by feeding our babies from the very first moment they open their eyes.

I didn't know any of this when I reached for the milk carton in my mom's fridge, but that's what I was looking for. Even my three-year-old daughter searches for my breast to find comfort, to get my attention, and to feel my caressing fingers on her back and neck. She looks for nourishment.

I was a shy little girl with a passion for color, horses, gymnastics and the 80s. I looked at adults as a different species than myself. My mom was my window to the world; anything else was bitter to me, including food. I drew a line separating my world and "theirs." My understanding of food was what my mother provided, what I ate at home. I can still recall the scent and taste of her dishes by just thinking about them. She would prepare spinach ravioli, parmesan hearts of palm, tomatoes stuffed with homemade mashed potatoes, steak stew, and spinach soup. Other than that, I was not interested in eating.

Vegetables were tough for me; I even disliked the sound they made when somebody ate them raw. Spinach was a special case, and that was only because Popeye, my favorite cartoon character, made me understand I needed spinach to be strong. Fish was repugnant – I couldn't stand the smell. I was grossed out by anyone eating roasted chicken on the bone in front of me, and if I ate it I would avoid smelling my hands afterwards because the smell stayed on my little fingers. I never liked red meat, though I ate it because it was what I understood as the fuel I needed to grow. Culturally, that was the message instilled in us in Colombia, but it would take me about twenty minutes to chew a piece of steak, and most likely it would end up thrown away in a paper napkin when nobody was looking. I did like hamburgers though, with ketchup.

Salsa de Tomate

My family, my grandparents and I had just arrived in the Dominican Republic. We were taking a vacation together far from the cold weather of Bogotá. We sat down by the hotel pool in the outside dining room feeling pretty hungry. We ordered hamburgers and French fries – this has become the universal food language for a kid. When the food arrrived, I asked for *Salsa de Tomate*. I could not eat unless I had some red sauce to smear on each fry. The waiter didn't know what I was talking about, even though we spoke the same language. I did my best to explain myself – "You know, tomato sauce." He laughed understandingly, nodded, and brought me four slices of tomato. Finally, we broke through the cultural gap and he brought me what he best knew as "ketchup!". Ketchup was the main vegetable during my years growing up; and sadly, to this day in our schools, it's still the main and only vegetable given to our kids in the form of pizza sauce or the highly processed Americanized version known worldwide as *ketchup*. Originally, ketchup was Chinese, and the word itself is a transliteration of the pronunciation of the Chinese word meaning "fish sauce".

Everywhere we traveled, there was the "burger and fries" and ketchup on the menu. We traveled every summer, mostly to Disney World. On these trips we ate at McDonald's and every other fast food chain there was. They spoke my language, they gave me *my food*, and on top of that, the "happy meal" came with a miniature plastic Barbie dressed in hot pink tights and *tulle* – back then, if you gave me a couple of those Barbies, I would eat as many hamburgers as you wanted. Meals became so easy during our travels, how could my parents ever question what was behind the white painted clown face that provided such convenience? Traveling to the States and going to their cleverly marketed and advertised stores meant only one thing to us; we can trust them, or so we assumed.

When we were in the States, everything had a sense of freshness and newness; it had a certain harmony even though it was loud and intense. Being a visually driven girl, as most kids are, I was fascinated with every single package, TV ad, or plastic toy that I saw. It was as if adults had broken the code and entered into my imaginary world to communicate directly with me. And there was no harm to it, or so we thought, because my parents, relying on their human naïveté, approved of them.

I wouldn't say I struggled with eating per se growing up. I just didn't like to eat just for the sake of food. I ate for what was around food, for what food represented or could bring to me in an existential realm: home, trust, and connection with my inner world. But I did not completely lack understanding of the other aspect of food; which is health. I had practiced gymnastics since I was one. I grew up doing gymnastics almost daily; my body was my instrument that turned in all the flips and spins I could ever dream of. Connecting with my body in this way at such a young age may have influenced me to take good care of it. I needed strength, so I ate spinach, or would down a glass of milk every morning because "healthy bones", or eat a hamburger because "meat" was the fuel I needed. In our Latin cultural understanding, that was what "nutrients" were.

"Nutrition" meant to do the right thing for my body. One day in first grade while still living in Bogotá, we had a group of people come to our class to talk about nutrition; they specifically talked about soda beverages and their harmful effect on our bodies. On that day at age 8 I made the decision to eradicate sodas completely from my life; to this day, it is a vow I am still keeping.

I always think back to this anecdote and reflect on my daughter. What kind of relationship with food am I inspiring in her? How am I presenting food to her? What are the values associated with food that I want to embed in her subconscious? Relating this event to my current life, my daughter has no recollection of what sodas, Coke, or Pepsi are. That day in my first grade class had a ripple effect which inspired me to do the right thing for my body and to pass on this principle to my own daughter. I'm teaching her about where food comes from, but as much as I have to do for her, I also have to "undo". We don't have a TV at home to avoid commercials and mainstream shows, though we can stream movies and narrow down our selection to the programs or movies we like to watch, in a way, we are choosing what information we want to feed ourselves.

It's in our Nature to trust one another. We go to the doctor, and although we have never seen him before and know little of him, we trust he is doing the best for our families. When we drive around the city, we trust that no car is going to purposely hit us. When we buy food, we trust what we are buying is safe for our kids. However, trust is now taking us farther from health, it's making us blind to the truth. In a way, that innate trust we have of others has become a form of ignorance. When it comes to the food we feed our children we must take the blinders off, because unfortunately the corporations that manufacture our highly processed and convenient foods are not in business for the sake of our kids' progress, but to make them into their loyal customers at an early age. Food ads are specially targeted to kids aged two and three for a reason. Once they hook a kid at that age, they will embed an emotional memory that will bind them to that food forever.

I belong to the information generation. Compared to our parents' time, especially growing up in a much more conservative third world country, living in Miami I now have access to knowledge that they never had. I can on google, buy books, attend seminars, and take online courses and classes in whatever topic I want to chocolate-dip-coat myself in. But information also comes with responsibility and the need to take action. I cannot just lecture my daughter about food, I can't sell her a concept that certain foods are "bad" or "good" – I must not skew her own curiosity about food – but I can show her by example how to honor, appreciate, and respect food, which is now my responsibility.

Back in my first grade classroom,, what spoke to me was the purity of the message: you can harm your body with sodas. That was all, there were not loud red fonts nor shiny packages. All the love invested in my gymnastics classes, the discipline my mom and I devoted to my practice, the positive feedback from my gymnastic instructor, and the freedom that I felt twisting like spaghetti and flipping like a monkey in the air shifted my thinking into respect for the choices that would impact my body. You see, my association with food back then, "nutrition," was linked not only to doing the right thing, but being "better".

[Burnt]
Mushroom Soup

Our brains started to expand the moment civilization discovered fire, because we began to cook! Fish was now part of our diet, and the inclusion of healthy omega fats and sea nutrients boosted our brain development and our thinking*. The one thing fish has in common with breast milk is the amount of fat. Breast milk is 90% fat, since it is intended to nourish our babies, and essential fatty acids are the main source of nutrition to help our kids' brains develop.

Cooking is a never ending play where Nature's elements, earth, air, fire and water, take main roles on the stage. The story that unfolds is mainly the interplay between ingredients and the chemical and cosmic reaction of the elements. The sensations it arouses wake up each of our senses. The transformation of the food from its raw stage to its final prepared state invites our sight. Cooking stimulates our sense of smell when the garlic melts in the pan, or when the fricassee vegetable casserole emits its special aroma. Our hearing alerts us to our next meal: the sound of oil sizzling on iron, the tempo of a chef's knife against the cutting board, or the singing of the fire outdoors. Cooking invites us to break bread, to feel the warmth released from the steaming lasagna, or to cool our throats with a frozen hibiscus lemonade. Cooking's flavors reach a peak in the mouth, relating each of our emotions and senses to taste buds that return bursts of *umami* euphoria.

Cooking is so much more than following a recipe; it requires our full attention and our unequivocal presence to perceive its alchemical transformation. It's about observing how long to leave the onion in the pan to caramelize, or how to use the tips of your fingers to pulverize the salt and just *feel* when the right pinch has been added. It's smelling the basil's sweet tones against the steam and letting our memory search for the right vinegar to complement it. Cooking brings you home, it grounds your feet to your roots. It connects you and nourishes your permanent awareness.

I have memories of cooking growing up. I am grateful that there was always food on the table. Whether we ate at grandma's, at home, or at my parents' friends' reunions, food was there. I don't even remember understanding the concept of a chef; it never crossed my mind that it could be a career.

---

* Origins Movie, Pedram Shojai

My closest understanding of someone that cooked was a woman on TV explaining how to make stuff step by step, I saw as a stay-at-home person, not a chef.

I remember my father making *aji* for the Sunday BBQs, or my mom preparing a taco buffet or her famous lasagna for house parties. But I didn't mess around in the kitchen till we came to Miami back in 2001. I was in my teens by then, but my curiosity for cooking came later, probably in my early twenties when I started experimenting with some recipes; however, my attempts met with failure time after time but I was missing the whole point of cooking.

I cooked out of fancy cook-books with photos that made your mouth water. I cooked with a watch to time the minutes listed on the recipe, and probably turned my back to the stove while waiting for the clock to beep. I would substitute ingredients, whatever I thought was the closest to what the recipe called for; I would add uneven amounts of flour that might or might not be what was listed on the cupcake recipe because I thought, what difference would it make? The result was always a burnt pan, a weird undercooked cupcake, or a burnt mushroom soup with red wine that tasted more like warm charred wine than anything else. I'd get furious. I was expecting magic to happen but the book lied. After several attempts, my family banned me from the kitchen, and I flipped my middle finger to cooking.

Back then my ingredients came in containers, but I never wondered where they originally came from. This is a fundamental question if you want to cook, because the story of the ingredients' origin carries little secrets about how it should be cooked, for how long, what its effect will be in a recipe, and what can you combine it with. I wanted instant transformation at the wiggle of a magic wand [or the touch of a button on the electric stove], but was missing that it's the cook who conducts the play, but the ingredients are the main actors on center stage. Once I understood that, cooking, became magic.

Chicken Nugget

I had my dark days when I moved to Miami. I felt like I didn't belong. The culture shock was painful. I felt frustrated living amongst people in my school who couldn't tell communists from community. Private school life had coated the kids' reality with fancy cars, sports, sex and drugs. Everything seemed like it was out of a mainstream American high school movie, all so pre-manufactured and methodical, so disconnected from the emotional aspects that need to be embraced in a teenager. It was all black or white. Even what they fed us complemented this confusing flat-thinking educational system: fried chicken nuggets, pizza, tomato sauce, and white bread. The food fed to us was so overprocessed and distant from its original source, as was the understanding of the school system as far as teenagers. I remember always asking, "What part of the chicken is a nugget?"

But not everything was so flavorless. I was fortunate enough to live next to the ocean, to meet people from all corners of the world, and to have the freedom to do things on my own I would never have been able to do back in Bogotá, like jogging around my 'hood at sunset.

I found a way to shift into a mentality that allowed me to explore Miami. But my hot-cold mood swings of mine landed me in the doctor's office. I was diagnosed with hyperthyroid, prescribed medication, and told I was destined to be on the pills the rest of my life, unless I decided to have my thyroid removed or radiated to ashes.

Why? Why a thyroid issue? Where does it come from? I couldn't get any answer that made sense. They said it could be genetic, or else that's just the way it is. I refused to accept the latter, because "just the way it is" meant to me that Nature had made a mistake; even with the little I knew, that was a concept I refused to accept. If there's one thing in our entire universe that's perfect, it's Nature.

Years later I found out that our thyroid hormone is extremely susceptible to stress. The stress response in our bodies calls us into our "fight or flight" response, wreaking havoc on our digestion and sending our hormones in all directions like popping corn. The thyroid is one of the main hormones that regulates our mood, energy levels, weight, and digestion. And it is bombarded daily by the masses of chemicals in our environment and in our household products, as well as the aluminum, fluoride and chloride found in our body and hair products and the preservatives and artificial hormones added to our foods. The endocrine system also is connected to balance from a mind-body psychological perspective. Could it be that feeling so out of whack in a new city and environment where I fought to belong had caused my hormonal and emotional self to fall into chaos and call for help?

Just the way it is? Huh.

I dropped the thyroid pills months after I started taking them. The whole thing didn't make sense to me, and since I could never see physical results of any kind, I simply forgot I had any sort of imbalance in my body. But my illness prevailed.

Cold Turkey

How you show up to the table is a reflection of how you are showing up to life. These are profound words by Marc David, founder of the Institute of Psychology of Eating and one of my mentors. How we show up to the table is a question we must ask ourselves to reevaluate not only our relationship with food, but also our relationship with ourselves.

Nowadays, we eat with the phone in one hand, in front of the computer, thinking about the next thing we have to do as soon as we unwrap the cold sandwich for lunch, and we eat in less than 15 minutes. No wonder we are so disconnected from our own humanity. All the advertising messages [including the subliminal messages] attempt to give us an instant answer, a band-aid for our problems. We all need to eat, of course, so then the answer is to squeeze calories and nutrients into a five-bite snack bar. How could we ever forget the fundamental principles that eating embodies? Actually, why are we not embracing eating and cooking as a family value, and as an act of self-love and respect? "A family that eats together, stays together."

Back then, I just didn't know better. I ate because I had to. I went to college because that's the way it was. I ate lean cold turkey with whole wheat bread because that was considered healthy back then. I ate for survival, but it was boring. I remember ordering a sandwich from the corner spot I usually frequented; since I didn't like food back then, I would speed-read the menu of twenty or so sandwiches that they had, roll my eyes, and then order the same thing every time. I got into a no-sugar fad and not for all the money in the world would I touch sugar. I drank my coffee black, and I completely lost my taste for baked goods or desserts.

I had studied fashion as a creative outlet on a rapid two-year college degree escapade. But though I am creative, it never really filled me up. I tried convincing myself to go with it, but it never worked out for me. In a way, you could say that I was eating but not being nourished, as I was working but not fulfilling my dreams.

I was living, but not living. I was there but not present. I was trying to fill a mold that didn't fit me. I was following a bland script. I was showing up to the table completely uninterested, and giving up the responsibility of searching for what represented true value for me.

Eggs and Bacon

Appetite for life! It's funny how many times we use this expression, without stopping for a minute to think that the food connotation here is no coincidence. How you do food is how you do life. It's established that we eat for survival;our appetite is a natural built-in mechanism that makes us respond to hunger either through cravings or a salivating mouth signaling us that we need to eat. There's nothing wrong with feeling hungry, it actually proves that you are longing for something. Though in our society we often punish ourselves for being hungry, that is as insane as asking us not to sweat. When you are hungry your body is talking to you. Looking behind the curtain of our appetite, being hungry means you are growing and expanding, it means you are alive, and it means you are demanding fuel to recharge the energy you require to thrive and act on what you are most passionate about. Having an appetite for life corresponds to happiness, to wanting to lengthen your life and enjoy every single day as the best day it can be. So, who's hungry?

He was a tall, blonde, green-eyed guy with a sweet voice and that Colorado swagger, half hippy, half surfer dude, that he had gathered from his various travels around the country. He was full of energy, always willing to help and to lend a hand. The life of the party. He loved to eat, but favored desserts above anything else. We fell in love. Together we road-tripped the country from coast to coast in his F150 truck, starting off with Burning Man in Black Rock City, Nevada, and returning three months later to Miami. During the trip I eased into his ways; we camped out most of the time, hiked and slept under the stars, and ate a whole lot of eggs and bacon. He was in charge of the cooking, because I sucked at it. I *could* fry an egg in a pan, but he went all fancy on me and broughta cast-iron skillet to cook with, and that was just odd, since I had never seen one before – and he wouldn't let me wash it.

But day after day camping on the road I became interested in what he brought to our "table." At first we had stack of dry goods, oatmeal, nut milks, beans, bread, and Nutella. We traveled chasing the fall, so the cooler temperatures helped conserve some of the groceries we would get in the city. I re-learned to eat by watching him eat. He had such a passion for a good meal, a cozy restaurant, and chocolate. We'd stop at local diners, or west coast "farm-to-table" restaurants he found on Yelp. He would go off about food trucks and how that was going to be the next big thing – and it was. His appetite basically rubbed off onto me, and I started to discover that food could taste good, that it was meant to be shared, and that food is a call for celebration.

Finally I started to make breakfast for him, using his beloved iron pan, over logs, dry branches and an open fire. There was something inside me that really always wanted to cook, and what better audience to try it out on than a guy who would eat burnt toast if it was offered to him!

During one of our adventures outside the Colorado Canyon, camping near buffalo under the bright light of the moon, it came to me. Out of the blue, I set up the menu for the night: broiled mushrooms stuffed with veggies. As if I knew what I was doing, I cut up the vegetables, cleaned the Portobello mushroom, stuffed it, packed it inside a foil pocket I had created, and threw it on the fire. For me, that was the first time I ever truly cooked. I was guided by my instinct, as every cook is. I was driven by the ingredients, the pitch-black cold night air, and the sound of the fire burning. In that moment, I felt as If I had cooked forever. It felt true. I felt that I was home.

Tofu

We reject what we need the most. We tend to turn our back on the things we need to listen to more deeply. If you asked me about vegans before 2010, I would have said they only ate tofu. I got the whole part about not killing any animals, but I just couldn't wrap my mind around why not eggs or dairy, if that didn't require any killing. I always asked people I knew who were vegan: Why? They would explain that it was a boycott of animal farming. That just sounded too complicated to me.

Before I became vegan I was lost and confused. Since I first began to have cognitive function, I've wanted to find my people. I wanted to find my tribe, but where was it, and what exactly did they look like? I was an atheist and a pessimist, I was angry at the world, I was missing a reason to believe in humanity.

After the road trip I started writing as a side job for different fashion publications. I had a friend and teacher who would mentor my grammar. JJ invited me to one of his literature classes. When I sat down in his classroom to watch a speech by Gary Yourofsky on the web, my world shook and changed forever. The video detailed the dark and cruel reality of factory farming involved in the industrial production of dairy, eggs, poultry, fish, and meat.

It was Nazi acts of violence and animal torture; I had not allowed myself to even wonder that such things could exist. Seeing in the video how the animals were disrespected, amputated while alive, humiliated, antibiotic-injected, and forced to overproduce in crowded filthy cages caused me to hurt all over. The video made me see how ignorant and irresponsible I had been in my own existence. I was buying and consuming out of convenience as many of us do, thinking that moderation is the way to be, when in fact it is pure mediocrity. I feel that we blind ourselves because it's easier. We turn our trust to familiar corporate brands instead of taking the responsibility of searching for small companies that truly care for our health outcomes.

This presentation gave me the sense of belonging I was longing for. It awoke in me the empathy for other living beings, and respect for those who are weaker than us. I wanted to be part of something that made existential sense; I needed to feel useful, to have a purpose. Veganism gave me a reason to make my choices in line with my values and to make my presence stronger; it opened a portal of transformation. I went vegan out of rebellion.

Fuck moderation.

Nourishing Path

- What does nutrition currently mean to you?
- What was your favorite food growing up and why? Can you relate your fascination with this food to who cooked it for you or where you ate it?
- Are you familiar with the ingredients you use, the brands you buy, and the companies you are supporting with your dollars?
- Are the meals you eat feeding you or nourishing you?

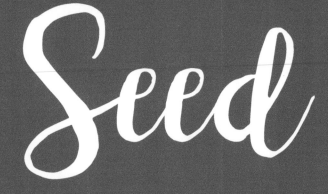

"Tal parece que en un extraño fenómeno de alquimia su ser se había disuelto en la salsa de las rosas, en el cuerpo de las codornices, en el vino y en cada uno de los olores de la comida."

— *Como Agua para Chocolate*, Laura Esquivel

Carob

"Adopt the pace of Nature: her secret is patience."

- Ralph Waldo Emerson

It takes time. We can't use the cold turkey approach to change a lifestyle from night to day. We can't beat a change out of ourselves. We can't force ourselves into doing better with punishment or pain. Life works in mysterious ways, and so does the body. It actually listens to us, and it's ready to speak when it needs to call for our attention.

We are too hard on ourselves. We always try to eradicate something in its entirety or expect an instant answer. Since becoming a vegan meant life to me, I took a different approach to it. I turned my rebellion into a creative force. I was charged. This was no punishment, but an act of love and power. So I made a deal with myself: I'd go completely vegan for two weeks, and if I felt fine after that, then I'd transition into dropping animal food groups one by one over time. It had begun. After those two weeks I was ecstatic. I dropped all chicken and turkey and dairy with the exception of Parmesan cheese or when eating brick oven pizza. I really wasn't eating red meat so that was simple to leave out. I still ate organic wild-caught fish and pastured free-range eggs, mainly because I had finally found a place to enjoy eating fish and crustaceans and also because it was a way to celebrate when eating out with my partner – but now I demanded quality.

I shifted myself into a vegan diet by falling in love with the act of eating. This is a fundamental principle at the table and in our lives. What pleasure brings to our bodies is far more chemically intricate than just a simple moment of euphoria. The pleasure of eating triggers a chemical compound called *colecystokinin*. Colecystokinin is responsible for stimulating the appetite in response to protein and fat consumption, turning on the metabolism, burning fat, and signalling your body to stop eating when you've had enough. It's the same compound that tells your cerebral cortex "it's pleasure time" so you can relax[*].

---

[*]   Emily Rosen https://www.youtube.com/watch?v=lE-A5OSsAX8

When eating out, the options on the menu narrowed down to the "sides" section, which made it easier to decide what to order. Trust me, the fewer options you have to choose from, the happier camper you'll be. If that wasn't the case I loved to heckle the waiter, making him or her squeeze a vegan dish out of the chef. I made every task that required an extra step mischievously pleasant. It was not always easy, but with the right attitude, everything is possible.

I went back to school, this time to pursue advertising, and lucky me, it was in the perfect location across from a friendly modern vegan empanada joint that sold veggie burgers with sweet potato fries and homemade ketchup as well as vegan soups and right next to it across the street was my new found paradise, Whole Foods.

My favorite thing to get there were those rice milk ice cream bars coated in a candy shell made of carob, a bean commonly used to replace chocolate. My meals were the highlight of my days. It was as if I had never had taste buds and now I had a whole fresh new set.

At home, we would usually eat out, so it was not a problem to choose my vegan foods and let him order his meat. I was not into forcing him to abandon his steak, as he was respectful of my new vegan ways.

Veganism taught me a beautiful lesson; in the midst of the radical political and ethical thinking, it showed me a new door to Nourishment and Pleasure. I never said to myself, "you have to be a full on vegan now," because it was no destination but my new path. I just felt like roaming over calm waters where I could sit back and experiment with foods. However, my priority became to really enjoy this new journey.

Decaf Coffee

"Nothing goes away until it teaches us what we need to know"

– Pema Chodron

It's not easy or natural to understand that something is wrong with one's body. You're never truly ready to deal with such a reality. I hadn't been diagnosed with any terminal disease, but the concept of having something wrong with my body, of accepting that I was "broken," didn't sit well with me.

My hands started to shake, and my heartbeat was elevated. My moon cycle was never regular. Those were the initial hyperthyroid symptoms I experienced, although I was never told the latter was related to the thyroid until later. I had very little tolerance for alcohol or coffee. So I switched to decaf. I later learned decaf is more acidic and more harmful to your gut than regular coffee. My mood would suddenly drop; I could become hysterical quite easily, or develop an uncontrollable need to cry. I had lost ten pounds when I switched my diet, and then lost ten pounds more due to my hyperthyroid condition.

Imbalance overpowered my life, work, relationships, and family. I returned to an endocrine doctor who ran more blood tests, and the results still showed my thyroid was overactive. The doctor's answer remained the same: take synthetic hormone pills for the rest of your life, or remove my thyroid. I couldn't go along with that.

My love relationship was not very stable. We would live in paradise while traveling and catching waves in Costa Rica, then we'd return to a hell surrounded by alcohol and drug demons. We lived in extremes, him with his addictions, and me with my hyper and erratic behavior and my fear of failure. When darkness surrounds your own shadows, it's difficult to break through and take the most fundamental action of survival: taking care of yourself. Refusing help or denying that one needs help is part of our human sickness, and when that happens, our own selves are our biggest enemy. It's a vicious cycle we simply want to remain trapped in. Getting help or reaching out of the swamp of depression meant "growing up", and that, my friends, is scary.

We made it through the dark tunnel somehow. I quit advertising school and decided to open a small fashion boutique in Wynwood. He slowed down a bit, and together we moved into a new apartment. One sunny Wednesday morning before getting ready for work, I sat down in our wooden porch to sip my cashew foam decaf coffee as usual and receiving an unusual call. Since my period was irregular, I had gone to the gynecologist to run more blood tests. I picked up the phone and it was the nurse telling me, "Pamela, you are pregnant."

I sank. I felt the wood underneath me melting. I was just in shock for several minutes. There was finally a reason for my extreme hormonal responses, shaking hands, and rapid heartbeat.. I panicked.

Love

First you think about everything that could go wrong. Where are we going to live, how am I going to work, will there be enough money, the future. I never wanted kids, why bring more innocent souls to this disastrous planet if we are all going to end up destroying our own? Or so I thought. However, there's a force of grace inside of me [and all of us] that spoke and guided me in the right direction.

In that moment it was that little soul that lit the way. She mattered above anything else. It was not about me anymore. I had life growing in my guts. Nothing else mattered. Not the money, not the pity problems of the everyday nor the past.

They say beauty is in the eye of the beholder. Well, they are right and they are wrong. Beauty is a feeling within the beholder inspired by purity, innocence, and raw love in what you see. I felt beautiful again because of her.

The reason to take care of my body was now transcendental. The seed that I carried in my womb planted a seed of its own in me, a seed of growth, maturity, expansion and evolution.

Hungry

My hyperthyroid condition had worsened until it bordered an autoimmune disease. The endocrinologist told me there was a risk of my baby dying at birth. He also said I would not be able to breast-feed ever and that there was no chance of a home birth. He prescribed me some pills to take and promised to lower the dose if I showed signs of recovery. I felt like I had my hands tied behind my back, I couldn't risk something happening to my child. I accepted the pills, but in the back of my head it drummed loud and clear, "I'm having a water home birth and I'm breast-feeding my baby!"

I dropped the gynecologist whose ideal of a perfect birth was a mother in a hospital bed watching TV with a remote control to auto-medicate an epidural for the contractions and pain. Soon after, I found a beautiful midwife-godmother who guided me through the pregnancy, although by law she was required to have me see a gynecologist due to my thyroid disorder. She introduced me to a doctor she worked closely with, but I didn't hit it off well with him either.

Meanwhile, I continued to search for the "other way". I googled diets, perfect foods to eat, vitamins to take, holistic ways to treat my thyroid, and it was all blank. Even the most basic information on how to be a new baby momma was so contradictory. One site would say to eat fish, while the other would say the mercury of the fish you are eating might be fatal to your baby. All I found was frustration.

The first three months were a nightmare. I would wake up hungry and nauseous, would eat and throw up right away, only to then be hungry again. I didn't like my doctors and I was afraid of what I could be doing to my child with the pills, but we had monthly ultrasounds to check her growth, and to my relief, she was doing fine.

Fear

Little do we know how much our bodies respond to our emotions, or that being sensitive is not a sign of weakness. We might complain, roll our eyes, or avoid eating with those with food sensitivities. But why don't we look a bit deeper? Being sensitive means we feel stronger and have a greater awareness than others; it means our hearts are more open and our intuition is better tuned. Having a food sensitivity simply means we are a tad extra developed and can feel the effects of external substances in a more acute manner. How many of us can smell aromas before others do? Or know that somebody is going to call, and then the phone rings? Back in the day, they called that witchcraft; nowadays I stand by it, and I might say I'm a bit of a witch myself. Being ultra-sensitive is my superpower.

Little do we know that being sensitive is linked directly to our hormones, especially the thyroid, which is the chief hormone in charge of regulating a plethora of systems in our bodies. When our mood, our lives, our financial stability, our love relationships, and even our self-love is at risk, our bodies will suffer and the thyroid may go berserk[*].

Every feeling of stress which is any real or imaginary threats you think you face will create a fear reaction in you. This fear attacks your gut, which can also be called your second brain, and can create a medical condition called hyper-permeable intestines, more commonly known as "leaky gut". This happens when your intestinal lining becomes porous, and then after you eat, the toxic substances your body is supposed to eliminate get sifted through the stomach lining and into your blood, reaching other organs. One of those, of course, is your thyroid gland.

Sensitive people are more susceptible to toxicity in the environment, whether physical or emotional. When you are stressed, it's not only your brain that suffers, but you are indeed stressing your organs as well. For those of us that suffer from thyroid issues, it's not for us to ask, "why me?" or to feel self-pity. It's the language of the universe communicating through our symptoms telling us that it's time to find balance.

No one is born with a bad thyroid or body. What we think are our weaknesses are simply a doorway to take advantage of our superpower.

---

[*]   Dr. Josh Axe https://www.facebook.com/DrJoshAxe/videos/10154440574306178/

Sunfoods

"The very first step before you begin a journey is an undiminished decision as to where you are headed."

– David Wolfe

I was hungry for information. It was a constant prayer, a rerun question that wouldn't go away, just as an earworm gets stuck in your head. Finally an answer came. I stumbled upon an advertising school friend who had dropped out after she got pregnant. She was now leading a movement called @VerdeYRebelde on Instagram. She had turned her life around and was now pursuing a career in functional nutrition and fitness. We chatted, and right away I knew that if I wanted answers, I had to dive deep into the issue. I followed her lead and completed a certification on holistic nutrition at the Institute of Integrative Nutrition.

I would come home from my store around eight in the evening, tune into the online school presentations, and eat; and then watch all kinds of food documentaries like "Hungry for Change", "Forks over Knives", or "Food Matters" on Netflix, or YouTube videos on holistic nutrition, or read books by David Wolfe.

All this information really woke me up, like a kick in the gut. Much of the time my jaw was dropping in awe or disappointment. I was getting tons of information, which was educational but also shocking. Our society recurs to western medicine doctors who treat the symptom not the problem. The US and New Zealand are the only countries in the whole wide world who allow televised ads for prescription drugs. The United States is the 37th country – next to Serbia – on the scale of the medical care system, isn't ironic to think, the US is one of the richest countries of the world, but also one of the sickest?. Splenda was discovered in 1976 while attempting to create a pesticide, yet that's what many of us mix with caffeine, chew in bubble gum, or chug in the form of diet Coke, creating a toxic environment that kills neurons by the second.[*]

---

[*] Hungry For A Change movie on Splenda

But the golden ticket, the answer to my prayers, the music to my ears was: The body can heal itself. Food is information and medicine. We can reverse any type of condition by eating a proper and balanced diet. A diet not only boils down to what foods we consume, it's about our life's philosophy and our lifestyle. In order to control your health, you have to control your ingredients; hence, you have to cook your own food. This was massive.

I learned from Joshua Rosenthal, founder of IIN, about the Macrobiotic lifestyle and mindset, which tells us that every action that we take with food affects the quality and nutritional value of the meal. Even transporting the food,washing it, every chop, slice, and even the cleanliness of the kitchen is a carried energy that is transmitted through the food. He encouraged us to prepare our own meals and to cook more often at home.

After him I encountered David Wolfe, a spark of energy who can light up the darkest amphitheater with his unstoppable shining knowledge. He would talk about raw foods, a completely new concept for me. He would break down not just the nutritional aspect of "sunfoods" – what he likes to call them – but also the healing and awakening power of every seed, nut, fruit, algae, mushroom and vegetable. He's addicted to the power of Nature, and I was addicted to what he had to say. "Food and Health are about Happiness."

Then it was the knowledge offered by Dr. Neal D. Barnard, a medical doctor and avid activist for plant-based diets, who merged nutrition with medicine in his practice as the ultimate prescription to help his patients.

After Dr. Barnard, Dr. Joel Fuhrman, more commonly known as the "Nutritarian", insistently taught that adults have to repair their bodies from the damage caused by our poor nutrition as kids. He says, "Most cancers are caused by what we fed our bodies between the ages of 1 and 10".

Then Andrea Beaman, chef and health counselor, talked about the importance of eating seasonally and maintaining a balance between yin and yang. She once suffered from thyroid disease and was able to reverse her body back to normal by balancing what she ate and the overall activities in her life.

Andrew Weill, physician and author, was also one of my favorites. He was not plant-based, but his approach to food was about respect and food's healing abilities. He introduced another new concept to me, that of the "Breath". I had never meditated or thought I could transcend anything by breathing, to me it was as unreachable as asking me to cook. But he explained how the breath is the master control of our autonomic nervous system, the link between our conscious and unconscious. Breathing can be an anti-anxiety practice and natural relaxer.

I continued to learn from experts in the field of holistic nutrition and functional medicine during the nutritional program. Some of the experts were in favor of a plant-based diet, some were vegetarian, and others were paleo or simply ate from all segments of the food chain. But the message was not about what regime to follow or what diet to stick to, the underlying link from one expert to the other was about food quality, organic, nutrient-dense foods, bio-individuality, a stress-free lifestyle, and *cooking* at home.

Faith

> "The single biggest thing you can do to take control of your health is cook."
>
> *–Jamie Oliver*

Wha is breathing without exhaling? Wha is eating without tasting? Wha is kissing without hugging? Wha is working without loving it? Wha is nutrition without faith?

The way you eat, the "diet" you choose, and the lifestyle you make for yourself say something about you. They express the way you see yourself, the way you value yourself, and the way you respect and trust yourself. The way you eat says a lot about what you believe in.

I didn't have to ask– can I cure myself? Can I balance my own hormones? I simply knew without doubt I was going to do it. I didn't attribute that power to myself personally, but had an underlying faith in the power and kindness of Mother Nature. If I could align myself with her greatness and adopt her pace and her wisdom, I trusted that I was going to make it. That's my definition of nourishment, the synergy between science and Nature, the bond between nutrition and faith. I started eating for nourishment with love and with a purpose, to provide the best vessel of growth for my daughter and to achieve balance and health for myself.

I cut out sugar since it's what feeds any type of virus, cancer or bacteria. I cut out gluten because it is linked to inflammation. I would only eat fish if a friend cooked it for me. One day, I decided to head to Barnes & Noble. I sat down in the vegetarian/diet section and spent about four hours going over recipe books. I took my time reading them and made sure that every book I bought had photos for almost every recipe; since I didn't want to be caught amongst fancy names or instructions, I wanted to be assured of what it was I was attempting to prepare.

My nightly routines now had two more chores added to them. Instead of ordering food in, I would cook from the recipe books, download a recipe from a blog, or follow a recipe from Instagram. My partner worked late nights, so when he came home, I would wake up and serve him up a homemade dinner and a baked dessert.

What's cooking without love?

Relaxation

"There's nothing like feeling alive to reset your stress levels"
–Pedram Shojai

Nutrient deficiency is probably the root cause of many illness and autoimmune conditions. However, it's not about the quantity of nutrients, it's about the quality and our mindset. Our mindset determines our nutrient assimilation, and the varied amount of vitamins and minerals already in our body will affect nutrient absorption.

When you show up to the table there's only two ways in which you can present yourself. Happy or Sad; Relaxed or Stressed; Joyous or Anxious, Alive or Zombie-Dead. This translates in your body to a sympathetic or parasympathetic response.

If you sit down to eat in a sympathetic response state, that is to say, if you sit down when you are stressed, anxious, angry, frustrated, sad, or in a rush, this is received as a threat to your body, and a number of symptoms that diminish your digestion's effectiveness are activated; it's like a domino effect[*]. This is the same "flight or fight" response found in Nature. When a gazelle feels threatened by a lion, her body instinctively turns on this response. The oxygen in the gastrointestinal blood flow rushes to her extremities so she can run for her life, her respiration increases, adrenaline is released to provide a burst of energy, and the digestive system (which is the system that requires the most energy to function) gets shut down completely. Digestive failure results in ineffective absorption of nutrients, nutrient excretion (via sweat or urination) and nutrient deficiency, a rise in cholesterol, salt retention, increased cortisol levels, and decreased intestinal flora and thyroid function, as well as turning off thermal efficiency, which is your ability to burn calories.

However, if you are a happy camper, and you sit down with an appetite for life, your parasympathetic response will rule your world, and every single system in your body will work harmoniously. This means your digestion is functioning fully, as is your capacity to burn calories, to absorb nutrients, and to relax.

I could have eaten the healthiest lunch every day, but without my presence and awareness at the moment of eating, I might as well have eaten junk. Our bodies respond to our thoughts, emotions, and belief systems. I aligned my thoughts with the purpose of healing myself.

---

[*]   The Slow Down Diet by Marc David, pg. 18

Maca

In my studies I came across maca, a superfood grown in the highest altitudes of Peru. It's considered an aphrodisiac and also an adaptogen. Years later I found out the true meaning of the term "adaptogenic", it describes superfoods or super herbs or medicinal mushrooms which when eaten convey the same tenacity the plant has to have in order to survive the harsh and extreme conditions in which it grows. Simply put, its ability to "adapt". Amazingly enough, just by observing the behavior and growth of a plant, one may be able to tell its healing qualities. This is a concept to digest and appreciate. This is the reason why eating organic is so important. This is what differentiates an organic apple from a pesticide-grown fruit. The quality of the crop is what makes the apple nutritious: the minerals present in the soil, the bacteria that helped provide food for the plant, the sun, the water, and the plant's growth process from seed to bloom. Just as the energy of a tortured animal remains in its tense nerves and is transmitted as information to our nervous system when we eat it, the same applies to the miracles of organic vegetables, fruits, herbs and mushrooms when we ingest them.

It turns out that maca directly influences the human endocrine system. "It provides hormone precursors that help the glands produce more and better-quality hormones and neurotransmitters"[*]. This is why it is highly recommended to assist the thyroid with adaptogens to support the stress tolerance levels in our bodies and aid in reaching balance. Back then I thought only this root had this effect, but its balancing qualities are also found in other types of adaptogens, like Reishi Mushroom, Chaga, and Ashwagandha, which is an herbal adaptogen that is great not only for thyroid imbalance, but for dealing with and adapting to stressful environments and situations and adrenal insufficiency.

I began starting every day with a green smoothie ritual. The smoothie consisted of baby greens, frozen pineapple, celery, coconut water, Maca, and spirulina. I also developed a great interest in seaweed at this time. Spirulina is a type of seaweed; next to hemp seeds and peas, it is the most concentrated source of plant protein. Since it's water-soluble as soon as it is ingested, our blood instantly absorbs it, in contrast to animal protein, which needs to be assimilated and requires much more energy to break

---

[*]   Longevity Now by David Wolfe, pg. 195

down. After the Hiroshima attack, survivors were able to battle the waves of radioactivity by consuming seaweed – one of Nature's foods that is richest in natural iodine, a mineral that assists the thyroid. Nori, the seaweed in which sushi is wrapped, is also a source of protein. Fast-forwarding to the present day, I pack nori as a snack in my daughter's lunchbox. You can toast it and salt it or simply buy it already toasted. It comes in different flavors and delivers an awesome powerhouse of nutrients in thin little crunchy paper-like "crackers". But patients with Hashimoto's thyroiditis should be aware that it is not recommended to consume iodine if you have this immune deficiency condition. Iodine is still quite the dilemma when treating autoimmune conditions as not everyone reacts the same way to the mineral.

I also dropped soy since it alters the hormones, especially the thyroid and estrogen levels. I ate it perhaps once a month; but if you eat soy, ask if it is organic –you must, it's one of the five most contaminated and genetically modified crops in the US. The best way to consume soy is in sporadic amounts, and the best sources are tempeh, which is cooked and fermented, miso paste, also fermented, and edamame, which is baby soy beans.

I learned to use mineral salt instead of table salt. These two are by far the most opposite foods that come from the same place. Mineral salt contains a surplus of minerals that are essential to balance our hormones, especially magnesium. At the other end of the spectrum there is "table salt", which starts as a mineral salt and has undergone a process stripping it of all its minerals to be sold to chemical companies. The salt that is left is a tasteless powder that is bleached and contains added sodium, chalk-calcium, and even sugar. Salt is a crystal and should be respected as such. It is also a fundamental component for cooking that acts as a magic element, bringing all flavors into harmony. You can add Pink Himalayan salt, Black salt from volcanic grounds, Kalahari Desert salt, or grey sea salt to your pantry and your cooking.

I included a side of raw greens with all my lunches and dinners. I remember not liking raw baby spinach at first, so my trick was to cut it into very tiny little ribbons, this way I could mix it up with whatever I was having and the spinach would go almost unnoticed. The trick with kale is to massage it with your hands using a tiny bit of olive oil, a pinch of salt, and some lemon juice. This helps to break down the fibers of the kale for those who like me are new to eating raw vegetables and find that dark leafy greens can be harsh on our stomachs. By massaging the kale with your hands and wilting it a bit, it is predigested for your belly.

I learned to cook quinoa. Just remember the ratio 1:2, one part grain to two parts water. The simplest way to cook it is to put it all in a sauce pan, turn the temperature to high and let it boil; then lower the temperature to "simmer" or the lowest setting, cover it, and cook for 20 minutes. Since legumes, nuts and grains were now my protein, I bought canned black beans, chickpeas, kidney beans, and all the varieties of organic legumes I could find and simply mixed them with the quinoa, adding ribboned greens and seared or roasted veggies. That was lunch or dinner.

I also learned to make butternut squash soup with cashew milk, and today it is still my favorite cream soup. I'd drizzle a pumpkin with coconut oil, add a pinch of sea salt and black pepper, and roast it for 45 minutes, then blend it with cashews and water. And in that way, recipe by recipe, cookbook by cookbook, I became familiar with cooking, and it became my hobby and my favorite thing to do.

Breastmilk

A concern started to run through me as milk started to flow through my mammary glands. The reason why the doctors had said I couldn't breast-feed was the prescription pills contaminating my milk. As I intended to have a natural birth, I dropped the pills as soon as the blood test came back and showed a drop of the hyperthyroid levels into balance. My family was furious. My grandmother called me from Colombia to tell me that if I had the baby at home without a doctor she would never speak to me again. They were all concerned about my health and the life of my baby, and I understood that. But as a woman, it was my right to give birth in the most natural possible way as my child deserved and to breast-feed her as a matter of principle. No one was going to take that right from me. It was my natural birthright and I intended to claim it.

I was scared, but I was committed to my decision. No hesitations. I took a risk, a leap of faith. The blood tests came back again after I had gone off the medication, and my thyroid had stabilized itself. Since we had been checking the progress of the baby monthly via sonogram, we could see her beautiful and perfect development. Now I had my shield and my sword: I had balanced my thyroid, my baby didn't show any sign of abnormalities, and I was now a warrior with a destiny written in stone. I would give birth to my daughter at home, in water, and would breast-feed her for as long as she wanted to continue to breast-feed.

I can't attribute my balance to one single thing. I cannot say that it was only nutrition. It was a combination of everything I was doing. It was my decision to embody myself and claim what was mine, motherhood. It was my being present and taking responsibility for my health. It was searching for that resonance to my soul: a plant based path. It was remembering that 8 year-old girl who sought to learn better nutrition. It was an act of love for my child to take those first steps into the kitchen. It was my labor of love, my quest for nourishment.

Violetta

"Let me baptize my soul with the help of
your waters"

- Ibeyi

It hadn't stopped raining since the night before, and it was the rain that soothed me through the window as I went through contractions all night, not even knowing that was what they were called. As we left for the gynecologists office for some final blood tests and to ask the doctor to sign a document so that the midwife could attend me, my midwife called me. "I got you, sister. I have seen what you've battled with to have your home birth and I believe in you." The doctor refused to sign the document authorizing it, but the midwife was in anyway.

We headed home to continue packing. We were moving to a new apartment the next week, and expected to have the baby at the new house. But when we got home, my water broke. The damned contractions were starting in. My legs felt like they were being chopped off to a chainsaw and my body started shivering every time the contractions kicked in. My back just couldn't support my weight – I felt like if I was being stabbed. My uterus and abdomen felt as heavy as a sack of stones. Gravity was my enemy.

My partner called Sheila the midwife and put me on to talk with her. "Breathe," she said, and helped me rhythmically inhale and exhale long enough to pace down my adrenaline and soothe my pain. She arrived, and I held onto my breath as if it were a drug with my eyes closed.

My partner lit candles and put on some Mozart while the midwife set up the pool of water where birthing would take place in a matter of breaths. I jumped into the pool. My territory.

I was in a feline dance, in a trance, in a space that felt like purple heavens.

I let my animal instincts guide me, and I befriended the contractions; they were just bringing me closer to her. Four hours later at 12:38 a.m., after three big pushes, Violetta Sky was home.

If we are capable of creating perfect little souls, everything is possible, my friends.

Nourishing Path

- How strongly do you feel about your "diet" or the way you eat?
- How often do you allow yourself to seek pleasure in food?
- Do you enjoy your regular daily meals?
- What's your superpower?
- What does "nourishment" mean to you?
- How often do you cook at home? Are you willing to start cooking more?

Nourishing Tips

- Buy an exotic type of mineral salt.
- Have a side of greens with every lunch and dinner.

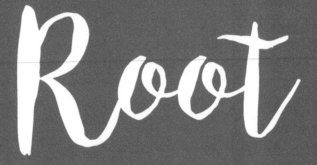

*"It was when I stopped searching for home within others
and lifted the foundation of home within myself
I found there were no roots more intimate
than those between a mind and body
that have decided to be whole"*

— Rupi Kaur

Coconut Water

We were stuck to each other. She was the size of my forearm. All she did was sleep or drink milk in her very first weeks of existence, or make little bubbles from her tiny lips, which I keep as treasured memories within my entire nervous system. I drank coconut water, and frankly, the first several days after the birth it was the only thing I had any appetite for.

Cravings. We might run away from them as if they were scary stalkers. But in fact, they are messages of information; besides symptoms, it's the other language our body uses to communicate with us. When we are craving something, we are craving much more than the substance itself. We may in fact be craving the feeling of a memory associated with the craved food, the sensation produced by consuming it, or the nutrients in the food. It is said that food is fuel, or that food is energy. Both are true. There are times when the body requires fuel to continue going, which is why it requires energetic foods to operate vibrantly and stay lively. However, food also serves our organs and all of our bodily systems as information, information that is decoded by our second brain – our stomach – primarily by our digestive system. When we crave food due to a nutritional deficiency, the body is telling us what system is in need of nourishment. I was craving coconut water due to the energy and vitality I expended during the birth. I was out of electrolytes and I needed to replenish my energies. Coconut water is Nature's best source of electrolytes. You may have heard of this, since coconut water is advertised with sports drinks.

Coconut Water replenishes the electrolytes and nutrients we sweat out during demanding exercise or movement, just as sports drinks do; however, the main difference between them is that one of them was fabricated by Mother Nature while the other is an attempt to mimic Her perfection. It's no coincidence that coconut water grows in the tropics and the hottest climates of our planet. Nature in her wisdom provides the residents of tropical climates an ambrosial beverage to help them survive depletion of minerals through sweat and heat. Just as every flower is conceived by a butterfly's proboscis, the food provided by Nature is designed to aid a specific cell or organ in our bodies.

After coconut water I wanted to eat chocolate, beans, and kale. Chocolate provides magnesium, which is an electrolyte as well. Magnesium helps to provide energy, calms the nervous system, regulates our sleep cycles, helps with digestion and constipation, and relaxes muscles[*]. Emotionally speaking, chocolate contains dopamine, which is a signal to our cells of calm, serenity, and relaxation. When stressed we often reach for comfort foods like pizza, bread, or pasta. This is due to the endorphins released when we eat these foods; in other words the body is craving relaxation and is asking us to slow down, sleep, and take your mind off whichever anxiety-producing situation you are stuck on. My reason for craving beans and kale was associated with iron and magnesium as well as other essential micronutrients.

What are you craving? Sometimes it can be as simple as wanting to remember someone. If you close your eyes and you think of eating your favorite dish as a kid, I bet you can still smell and taste it, and it takes you right back to the moment you enjoyed that dish, back to the music or the silence, the ambiance or the moonlight, those present and your feeling of satiation, love, and contentment. Sometimes, that's exactly what we are craving...

---

[*] https://draxe.com/magnesium-supplements/

Placenta Pills

Maybe the best gifts anyone can give a new mom are space and food. Space is respect for our animal instincts and momma bear feelings. It's a bond that continues to be woven between mother and child after the umbilical cord is cut off. Just as you wouldn't mess with a lioness in the wild when she just gave birth and shouldn't attempt to pick up her cub, or take it away from her side, you shouldn't do anything like that around any human baby momma either. Just my two cents...

Food. I was exhausted and weak. If only I had someone who could cook for me or bring me food. In these moments of nostalgia and euphoria after the birth, moms also need to be nourished. We go through so much pain, between the milk accumulated in our breasts making them rock hard and heavy, our sore cut nipples, and the wild time our hormones are having with our moods.

Luckily, my midwife had recommended eating my own placenta. She told me stories about moms frying it, or blending it and drinking it, and although I wasn't into doing it raw, I had my placenta picked up by another midwife who dried and pulverized it and gave it back to me in the form of capsules. I always look to Nature to understand what's natural for us. Every mammalian mother after delivering her pups or cubs eats the placenta. The theory behind this relies on supplying back to the body all nutrients that lost during birth. It also helps to enrich a mother's milk and in coping with postpartum and baby blues... This is truly being nourished by Nature.

Now I cook professionally for other new moms and deliver batches of food to them during their first days after birth. Funny how things come full circle. It touches me when the food I prepare is seen as sacred and necessary to nourish other souls.

Chocolate Oat Cookie

I never thought I was going to cook for a living. I didn't even imagine I was going to pursue cooking after giving birth. We were living a different life, now that I had a baby girl to look after, and I simply didn't see myself having enough time in the day to be able to spend it in the kitchen.

But the barriers we build around ourselves are probably the most difficult to dismantle; the image we have about who we are in society, who we are meant to be, and our purpose. I had it all wrong. I still owned my store, and it was open while I stayed home on maternity leave. But even when I was ready to go back, I didn't want to. I went into resistance about it. I started questioning the purpose of it all. I wanted to quit fashion, all of it, but what would become of me? A stay-home-mom, soon-to-be-housewife-and-childbearing-machine for the rest of my life? I feared not having a purpose, a service to offer, or a profession.

Meanwhile, to distract myself from my anxious thinking, while Violetta slept I would google new recipes and bake cookies during her naps. I would smile to myself, thinking I might be giving her "sweet dreams", since she would sleep while the aromas of vanilla, oats, and chocolate coming out of the kitchen would infuse the whole entire house.

Gut

Out of the blue, into the blue, while strolling around the neighborhood with my daughter an impulsive thought came to mind. I called my mom right away and told her I was going to close the store and wanted nothing more to do with fashion. It was something I hadn't wanted to let go of before, but now I did it cold turkey. I had no idea what was going to become of me; the vegan café where I was working couldn't afford me full time, and I didn't feel qualified to apply to any other restaurant. Also I would not leave my daughter for longer than four hours a day. I just faced my fear of the unknown and took the step anyway.

It was a gut feeling. It was as much impulse as intuition that made me decide to move on.

I like to think I'm an intuitive person. Some time ago, I thought that was just a talent certain people had, but it's not. We are all genetically equipped with intuition, or better said with gut intelligence, but some of us use that power more than others. The butterflies that we have all experienced in extra exciting situations or when facing fear are not just sensations without a cause. There is a biochemical explanation for them, and they are as real as when you experience pain from a cut that you can see on your physical body. Recently scientists discovered we have another nervous system called the enteric. It's a network of neurons and neurotransmitters that embrace our digestive organs, from our esophagus all the way down to our intestines. Studies have proven we have even more neurons and neurotransmitters in our gut that we do in our spinal cord. Therefore, the gut has been hailed as the "second brain" or the "gut brain". Our gut brain actually produces the same chemical substances as our head-brain, like serotonin and dopamine, and sensations of euphoria that we thought were produced solely by the brain have now been found to be in our stomach as well.

So when you feel those butterflies, when you get that hunch, you better believe it – your stomach is talking to you, and it may know better than your brain what the best choice is, who to trust, and of course what food to eat.[*]

Maybe is not that I'm such an intuitive person, but the truth is I'm more of a gut thinker than a brain listener. Aren't we all?

---

[*] http://psychologyofeating.com/the-brain-in-the-belly/

Mango Custard

"Success means we go to sleep at night knowing that our
talents and abilities were used in a way that served others."

– *Marianne Williamson, A Return to Love*

Above my computer desk I have a reminder that goes, "Our happiness and our function are one."* This is the challenge for a 19-year-old about to graduate from high school. We bang our heads against the wall asking for a sign of which path we should choose. We want to figure it all out right then by picking a career to determine the rest of our lives, as if at 18 or 19 we were savvy enough to understand the world, to know ourselves, and to comprehend that our lives have meaning that has nothing to do with how much money we will be banking in the future. "You are in business to spread love." Marianne Williamson further explains on her book *A Return to Love*, when talking about our purpose and careers. This might sound a bit idealistic, but I'm not anti-money or anti-wealth, I'm pro-abundance, and money should be seen as an extra abundance bonus that comes to you when you are expressing your gifts. Therefore, making money is not the end goal, it's a reward; however finding your purpose and contributing to the evolution of our species and the health of our community should be your focus, then the reward will come.

How many people do you know who are ecstatic to wake up early and head to their office? Or who after an 18-hour work day can still say, "I love what I do"? There is authenticity in these words; they are selfless and profound. I don't deny we like to make ourselves happy by going shopping, getting a new haircut, or taking a vacation. However, if that happiness is not be shared, eventually the magic of these adventures is lost. What makes our happiness eternal is the ability to share it and extend it to others. After all, we were given the gift of loving and being loved, and if it's not put into use, it's a lost life

The perfection of the Universe and Nature have also given us other sets of skills and different kinds of intelligence. Some of us are lucky enough to have these developed at an early age and by age 10 years,, already know what our destiny is all about. Others struggle, hopping from field to field trying to find what makes their heart sing and not settling until they do. Still others think that they lack any type of ability and just

---

* A Course in Miracles

go through the monotonous motions of working a job, getting paid, and sleeping. I don't think I'm special, but I've learned to differentiate between that state and being awake. We are all special, and so none of us are as well. I always thought, if another human being is capable of building a rocket ship, why can't I? At the end we have the same biology, circulatory system, and heart. But it's simply not what I came here to do, and thank God we are such a versatile population; once I decided to shake myself out of my comfort zone and wake up into my true rhythm, I realized that my function is to nourish the world. That's what I love.

When I started cooking I was unaware of that, but the impulse felt so pure and so natural that it was inviting to pursue it. With fashion on the other hand, I kept hitting bumpy roads and closed doors – signs that said, "look in another direction". When you are aligned with your path, life, the universe, God or whatever you want to call it, helps and guidance come to you. Your career is not separate from your daily life, but an extension of you[*]. There are people who come to this world to protect, to build, to teach, or to entertain. I came to wake up the collective consciousness of our humanity and invite us to live in unity and Harmony with Nature.

An enlightened path doesn't mean a flawless, white porcelain road. You will always encounter bumps, problems, and uncomfortable situations. What makes your path an enlightened one is your ability to see these difficulties as challenges and potential solutions to help you learn, grow, and keep progressing. It's all about changing your perspective!

After I quit my fashion career, a friend put me in contact with her chef boyfriend who was opening a new restaurant. His concept was a completely gluten-free menu and bar, however, it was not vegan. Since it was gluten-free, I felt I could work in the pastry section and avoid dealing with working with the butchering.

The chef was recognized in our city for honoring Miami's tropical fruits and for his Grandma's famous *Mango Pie recipe*. Hearing about his take on southern cuisine and sourcing of local produce made me feel safe enough to try a job in a non-vegetarian setting.

I had no clue about the business monster I was about to encounter. The restaurant industry is quite mesmerizing. Like a mermaid, it is attractive and seems romantic, but once you are entangled in her trap, the mermaid turns into a spider who binds you in her web and sucks you dry. You either love it or you hate it.

Working at this restaurant was a boot camp. I learned fundamental restaurant skills there, and now I thank them for my schooling. The Chef de Cuisine was on my ass all the time. She demanded perfection from every one of the items I "prepped". I thought she was crazy. But she was right. I just didn't know. I failed at dealing with gelatin, then gagged while cracking eggs, and I almost cried when I went into the walk-in cooler only to see a bunch of plucked and skinned ducks hanging there dripping blood. But all these obstacles empowered me. I had fallen in love with cooking, and I aligned my vision towards understanding what type of cook I was and what career I wanted to pursue. I was on a path to becoming a plant-based chef. As a plant-based chef, I would demand respect for the food and ingredients we use, quality at all times, and an attitude of service when preparing food, where every time I step into the kitchen I know that I'm nourishing the world.

Are your happiness and function one?

Are you expressing your love?

---

[*] Marianne Williamson, A Return to Love, pg. 179

Gluten-Free

"Our species as human beings will not survive, if we continue to destroy Nature."

– Bernie Sanders

What is it about gluten? I get a lot of my friends asking me about gluten and about the trend that rules our hashtags and social media accounts these days: #glutenfree. Should we go that route, or is this just a passing fad? I believe it's not a fad, and that the longer we continue to purchase gluten in processed foods and consume it, the more the wave will build into a tsunami of gluten-free-for-all. Almost every autoimmune condition known to man is associated with gut health. 80% of our immune system lives in our intestines, and the lack of proper digestion, impediments to nutrient absorption, and the permeability of our intestinal walls are the perfect storm for developing autoimmune conditions.

Gluten is a protein found in wheat, rye, spelt, and barley. We eat it in the form of pasta, bread, baked goods, and cookies, as well as in warm sauces and some salad dressings. The protein is what makes the flour sticky and useful for making delicious, self-rising biscuits and breads. It is the binding agent in flour. Once a short grass used in artisan bakeries, it is now one of the most genetically modified ingredients in the US, next to canola, soy, and corn. It's been modified now to be a tall grass in order to guarantee the self-rising factor, the binding properties of the flour, and even everlasting baked goods at your grocery store. Proteins are the most difficult substances to digest, and gluten is no an exception. When we consume low quality processed gluten on a daily basis three to four times a day, we are wreaking havoc on our digestive engine and causing a great deal of distress in our gut and intestinal wall. When this occurs after years of eating the same way, our intestinal impermeability starts to give up, and we end up with IBS, bloating, gas, allergies, skin rashes, fatigue, headaches – to sum it all up, what is known as leaky gut.

Leaky gut is when the wall that protects the gut becomes permeable. Think of this wall that surrounds your intestines as an array of red theater curtains hanging next to each other. When they are fully closed, they protect you from any pathogens outside of your gut and keeping indigestible substances inside your intestines to then excrete them via your colon. However, when the curtains start to open due to inflammation, and the gap between one curtain and the other becomes wider, it leaves space for all the toxins and bad bacteria, to travel in and out of your gut and into your blood. The toxins then are flushed to all major organs, your heart, liver, pancreas, glands, and thyroid.

When we have a substance in our stomach that is as hard to digest as gluten and we keep eating it over and over again, it stars to accumulate and create agony in the gut. If you don't have a condition known as celiac disease, which is clinically an allergy to gluten, you will develop sensitivity to gluten by eating low quality gluten in excessive amounts. This creates inflammation every time you eat it, and ongoing inflammation causes stress in the body. Stress triggers the release of another set of hormones and substances to treat the inflamed area, resulting in a never-ending cycle of inflammation and depletion of your body.

Whether you have a sensitivity to gluten or not, it's better to choose naturally gluten free grains like amaranth, rice, quinoa, millet, sorghum, oats, buckwheat, and chickpea flour, and only eat gluten on special occasions or when you find an artisanal stone-ground bread at the farmers' market. You can also eat naturally fermented sourdough, since during the fermentation of the dough, the yeast eats the gluten, making the bread easier to digest. Eat gluten only as the exception, not the rule. However, if you have an autoimmune condition or feel discomfort after eating gluten, leave it out. And to my thyroid comrades, gluten can really affect the levels of antibodies in your glands.[*] If you suffer from any thyroid imbalance, especially Hashimoto's, it's better to abstain from eating gluten, at least until you reverse your condition. Cutting gluten out can actually return your body back to health if that was the root cause of your autoimmune condition.

As you move into the kitchen, if you wish to follow a gluten-free recipe and you don't have the flour that was called for, do not just try to replace it with whatever you have in your pantry, especially if you are baking. Baking is a very exact art, and different flours have distinct characteristics. Each flour has different qualities; some of them naturally bind, while others can dry out the batter or will not bind or rise at all. Gluten-free baking may seem difficult to some because they are used to using only one naturally rising and binding flour, but it's not difficult, it just requires getting out of your comfort zone and being willing to do some experimenting. When baking gluten-free you must blend flours, add binding agents like xanthan gum, starches, or flax and chia meal, and become familiar with the properties of the flours. One awesome exercise is to get all your flours out and simply touch them and feel each one between your fingers; you will experience the difference in the grain texture and size, and you'll be able to *feel* its cooking properties. This will help you understand the behavior of each type of flour.

As I write this chapter, this morning I received the results of a sensitivity blood test. It turns out I'm sensitive to all dairy and eggs and can somewhat tolerate gluten, but can't have pineapple or almonds at all. Test or no test, the best indicator of your allergies and sensitivities is *you*. I guess I've been gravitating towards a vegan diet for a reason after all. Listen to your body, notice if there is discomfort and know that pain is not the way you should naturally feel at all. Your body was designed to thrive, and if that vitality is not what you are experiencing, then seek what may be causing its dysfunction.

---

[*] Root Cause by Izabella Wents, pg. 145

Umami

> "The doctor of the future will give no medication, but will interest his patients in the care of the human frame, diet and in the cause and prevention of disease."
>
> *- Thomas Edison*

What if in the future a chef's services can be included in your medical insurance bill? What if they teach cooking as a required basic skill in school? What if there was a mandatory one-hour lunch break for all corporate jobs? What if cooking and sitting together to eat could again become a family value that is passed on through the generations?

There's so much history in cooking, the ways grandma used to make things that get passed on to her grandchildren, the reasons why she picked certain herbs or used certain fruits – which has nothing to do with store-bought commodities, but with seasons, weather, economics, family, technology, tools, and ingredients. The plate tells a story, it collects memories; it's a reflection of our lifestyle.

If disease starts in the gut, wouldn't you say the foods you eat should be the primary focus of recovery? Even before sickness occurs, shouldn't the way you eat help to ensure you have a strong healthy body that can fight off viruses and cancers? It is a given that we are not invincible. Genetically we are prone to certain diseases, and due to the stress levels in our society, disease is certainly happening – 80% of our chronic issues are associated with the high levels of stress we are confronting nowadays[*]. But if we were nourished from birth and given wholesome foods during our childhood, if we banned GMOs and toxic chemicals from our crops and foods, limited the amount of processed foods in the grocery store aisles, reduced white sugar and table salt consumption, and increased our awareness of healthy and organic eating, then the medical bills will fall, and collectively we will understand that food is indeed our medicine as Hippocrates once said.

---

[*] The 3-Season Diet, John Douillard, pg. 5

"Give a man a fish, and he has a meal; teach him how to fish and he is fed for life," as the saying goes. I propose, "Teach a kid to cook, and he is nourished for life!" Cooking is a survival skill, just as making a fire and swim, and learning it is as essential as learning to read. If we don't take responsibility for our bodies, then we are passing the right to make our life decisions to others who will gladly take it on – for a price, of course. "They" will sell you a pill, and then another pill, the side effects of which then require yet another pill. "They" will sell you microwaveable trays of life-lacking foods. "They" will trick you into thinking that Coke Zero has no ill effects on you, that they have rediscovered the wheel with the invention of *Splenda* and drinks with zero calories per sip. "They" are just a reflection of "us". The more we give up our responsibility to take care of our bodies, to connect with our own inner selves and Nature, and to listen to our second brain and acknowledge its existence, the more we are voting for the party that encourages our lack of effort and lack of enthusiasm for living. "They" will hand us survival in a box with a price tag. So I say again, let's get back to the kitchen!

Cooking is more than a chore. It's not just one more thing you have to do, it's an activity you *get to* enjoy. We can all cook, no matter your background, your passions, or your past failures in the kitchen. If you can choose what to wear, if you know what music you enjoy, if you are able to make choices for yourself, then you can make choices in the kitchen. We all have a different hand when it comes to cooking; some of us have a heavy hand with seasonings while others have a delicate touch. If you are an individual who likes to eat, likes food, and you are capable of loving, then you can cook.

Cooking is a transformational act of love.

None of us were born with learned skills. We were born with different kinds of intelligence, and in the course of our lives we decided to develop some more than others. But someone had to give us some basic understanding of the various arts. Things would taste so much better if in school, science class could've dedicated a year to the binding and combining of flavors, digging into the different sours, sweets, fats, and salts that when combined create that *umami* sensation. Being able to cook takes some fundamentals, just as to know how to multiply you need to have learned how to count first.

Sugar

Around the 1960s the US government raised the question of health. One of the presidents at the time suffered a heart attack. Science tried to explain the root cause of his heart stopping, and they related it to diet. What came was blamed in that instance was "fat". However, at the time science didn't differentiate between the different types of fats, so the solution the US government came up with was to cut fat out of the diet. This inspired companies to create "fat-free", "reduced fat", and "low fat" products, and we became obsessed with calories. This was the historical moment when the calories in a food were required to be listed on every food label[*]. It was the craze of the moment. Many food corporations went with it and tried to create the magic fat-free low-calorie snack. But here's the trick: in order for a snack type food product to taste good, it needs fat, so the fat it gets replaced with sugar in order to appeal to the masses' taste buds. What happened after the late 1970s was an epidemic of obesity, diabetes, and other chronic illnesses that we are still facing today. 55% of the adult population is overweight or obese, and 22% of our kids are also suffering from overweight issues, a number that has doubled since the 1980s.[**] This fat reduction wave also introduced the number one toxic nutritional belief that has enslaved our bodies and robbed us of our happiness: FAT is BAD, furthermore, if I'm fat I'm not accepted. If I eat I'm getting FAT, and all FAT is bad.

Fat is not what makes us fat. Healthy fats, which range from saturated fats like coconut oil, palm oil, and butter, to monounsaturated fats like avocadoes and olives, and/or polyunsaturated fats like hemp seed, are fats high in Omega-3s, which also contain Omega-6s and Omega-9s. These fats are called essential fatty acids because they are necessary for our survival and proper physical function. Fat in our bodies is responsible for the health of our skin, hair, and nails; it regulates our mood, energy, appetite, and ability to lose weight, it protects our cells from malign substances, and it coats pathogen cells to protect us from their poisonous qualities. In women, healthy fats are what regulates our moon cycle and keeps our reproductive health in balance. For proper health, we want to keep a ratio of 1:1 of Omega-3s to Omega-6s. Omega-6s are the most common form of fat found in junk food, processed foods, and red meat. Omega-6 is also an inflammatory fat, which is the reason why we want to steer away from Omega-6 as much as possible and eat more Omega-3 rich foods.

---

[*]   The 3-Season Diet, John Douillard, pg. 27
[**]   The 3-Season Diet, John Douillard, pg. 3

Avoid cooking with any hydrogenated vegetable oil or buying products that contain hydrogenated oils; most boxed baked goods, cookies, breads, doughnuts, and baked kids' snacks contain them. Hydrogenated oil was the response of science to our fat scare epidemic. Their intention was to replace saturated fats like butter by taking a polyunsaturated vegetable oil through a synthetic process of adding hydrogen to make it solid at room temperature, resulting in a spread that mimicked butter known as "margarine". Furthermore, science was able to keep the vegetable oil liquid after hydrogenation so that it could be used in baked goods recipes, with the sole purpose of longer shelf life. These hydrogenated oils are what are known as "trans fats," and they are highly damaging to our bodies, arteries, and overall health.*

Vegetable oils like canola, sunflower, soy, and corn have little resistance to heat and become rancid when in contact with high temperatures. Cook with saturated fats, which are more stable and provide vitamins and minerals at the same time, such as coconut oil, palm oil – if it was sustainably harvested – and ghee or butter when farmed responsibly.

What creates fat in the body is sugar. Sugar is composed of two molecules called fructose and glucose. Glucose is the sugar found in carbohydrates and is food for our cells transformed into energy. The excess of glucose is then stored in the liver for when the body needs an extra resource. When glucose is present in our blood, the pancreas releases insulin to help our cells cope with the sugar and transform it into useful fuel. Fructose is the other type of sugar found in fruit, vegetables, sugarcane, and honey. When there are overwhelming amounts of fructose, sugar is then stored as fat throughout our bodies**.

Sugar, or a sweet flavor on our tongues, is also responsible for stimulating our digestive systems. At the first taste of "sweet" in our bodies, the insulin hormone is secreted to assist in the delivery of sugar to our cells, where it is then turned into energy. Please be wary of any type of "diet" product in the market – if you ask me, they should be labeled "nutritionally depleted". All the attempts to replace white sugar with synthetic sweeteners such as aspartame (a stimulant) and saccharine (a carcinogen)***can only cause harm and increase dependency on refined sugar itself. Abuse of these substances can also cause you to end up diabetic as insulin is released in vain, or to become hypoglycemic and dependent on a fake sugar rush, or to have further cardiac problems. *Please abstain from any synthetic substance!*

In babies and elders, sweetness is the predominant sensation on the tongue. It's the first taste to develop when you are young, and it's the last one to go in your last years. Could this be because enjoying food actually stimulates a biochemical response in our bodies, making pleasure when eating necessary? The answer is yes. But we will discuss that farther down, in the Root section. After establishing the chemical properties of sugar and understanding that the excess of sugar is what's harmful, let's dive in into its basic character. Simply put, sugar is a sweet flavor necessary to balance and give character to certain recipes.

Besides fat and sugar, to make a dish pleasing we need salt, an acid or sour, and a flavor profile, which can be spicy/pungent/herbal/earthy. I called those *cooking elements* or *kitchen elements*. I have my kitchen pantry organized by these elements, it makes my life easier when I'm cooking. I know that if I need to reach for an acid, I can turn to my vinegar section, and then my intuitive hunch feeling, or 'second brain', which is another tool in my kitchen, can decide which one to use.

---

*   The 3-Season Diet, John Douillard, pg. 29
**   Root Cause, Izabella Wentz, pg. 283
*** The 3-Season Diet, John Douillard, pg. 30

Cooking Elements

Fat: coconut oil, avocado oil, macadamia oil, sesame oil, peanut oil, palm oil, olive oil, melted cacao butter, or any cold-pressed nut or seed oil. It could also be any nut or seed blended into a butter, like cashew butter, peanut butter, almond butter, hazelnut butter, sesame butter, sunflower butter, or just the whole nut and/or seed.

Sugar: can be fruit or dry fruit, like apricots, prunes, raisins, dates, or natural maple syrup, coconut sugar or nectar, yacon syrup, honey, monk fruit, stevia or sugar cane. When making a savory dish, onions or garlic can be the sweet element of the dish, or perhaps the vegetable/fruit itself, like tomatoes, sweet potatoes, or even the same nut used for fat; or the type of vinegar can also add sweetness to your recipe.

Salt: can be pink salt, sea salt, flavored mineral salt, seaweed, tamari, miso paste, coconut aminos, olives or caper juice.

Acid/sour: can be any form of vinegar, such as apple cider vinegar, rice vinegar, white wine vinegar, red wine vinegar, plum vinegar, balsamic or white balsamic vinegar; you could also use citrus juice, or the juice of fermented foods like sauerkraut, kimchi, coconut kefir, or yogurt.

Lastly, the *seasoning* and *spices* will determine the flavor direction of the dish; possibilities include: lavender, chipotle, cardamom, cinnamon, turmeric, smoked paprika, vanilla, chocolate, salted caramel, ginger, and truffle oil! And the list goes on and on.

Just as corporations had to introduce sugar in place of fat to make their products palatable, we have to play around with the cooking elements to make our dishes pleasant to our taste buds. It's when we have a harmonious fat/acid/sugar/salt combination that pleasure arises in culinary terms.

Although sugar is necessary for some recipes, it's not essential for every single dish. However, salt is the number one component in your kitchen. You always want to have salt handy, as it goes in every single dish with very minor exceptions, whether you are preparing a dessert, a pie, or even ice cream. Salt is what brings the flavors into harmony. Don't be afraid to use mineral, which is not to be confused with table salt, as explained in an earlier chapter.

The best way to learn how to balance flavors is by smelling and tasting what you are cooking every time you introduce a new ingredient into the pot. This way you can wake up your dormant tongue intelligence and understand the *cooking elements.* This practice will show you how each ingredient reacts to the presence of others, how it is perceived by your senses, and how it chemically affects the end product. Another suggestion I have for you is to have fun at the grocery store – try picking one new flavored vinegar, oil, or spice and substitute it for what you have always used before. Start creating a beautiful collection of kitchen elements to play *witch* with when dinnertime is coming (or magician, I've also been called that at some of my dinner events).

Meatless Monday

"World peace starts in the kitchen"

- a T-shirt.

Vegetarians are boring. They only eat salads and raw vegetables. This is the number one misconception of what plant-based cuisine can be. Beautiful art is not merely associated with particular ingredients or tools, but also with aesthetic execution. A chef, who is an artist, should be able to deliver a delicious plant-based meal, just as he or she can perfectly sear a steak. The difference between good and great is in the execution. Execution also means the process of creation, and in order to create, one needs inspiration, passion, fire within, and a drive to want to perceive things in a different light.

In most kitchens, vegan or vegetarian dishes are not respected, as if making such plates is less than real cooking, boring, expected, and limited, when in fact it's simply a new approach to cooking. What most people don't know, however, is that plant-based cuisine is an elevated art that requires much more than just cooking skills. Plant-based cuisine presents us with a challenge and an invitation. The beauty of this type of culinary art is in the connection between the artists and their tools.

The tools of a plant-based chef go beyond the surface of the kitchen counter. Our tools and ingredients involve time, quality, the weather, the seasons, the four elements, and the entire living ecosystem. Our cooking is about life. We eat and work with the greatest expressions of Nature: plants, grains, seeds, flowers, stems, leaves, seaweed, mushrooms, and microbes. Our cooking is about awareness, connection, slowing down, observing, presence, and respect. Plant-based cooking develops your values and morals, and makes you a more conscious human being. Plant-based cuisine is an invitation to appreciate life in all its varieties, no matter how insignificant they may appear to be; and as the practice of yoga teaches us, cooking in this way invites us to take this philosophy into the wider arena of our lives, where respect for others, no matter their race, background, education, or religion inclination, is fundamental.

I have never met a plant-based eater that lacks a desire to make this planet a better place. It's a selfless practice. Once the decision to transcend into this lifestyle has been made, there's a deeper meaning, a fire burning inside, that brings each of us to revolutionize our lives.

Some people transition into a plant-based diet for health reasons, others in an effort to halt rapid climate change, others for political reasons, to boycott factory farming, cruelty to animals, and to stand up for animal rights, or to cultivate kindness. Being a vegetarian is not only a diet, it's a way of life, and its aim is to find harmony between our fast-paced city lives and Nature.

"Kill them with kindness" they say. I suggest, "Nourish them with kindness". That's the challenge, and the passion beneath our plant-based culinary art. We aren't trying to promote restrictive measures, but options that can enrich and simplify our lives. All the answers, all the antidotes to our suffering, are found in Nature and are available to all of us. Changing the way we eat is the first step to tapping into that energy, to becoming lighter and more receptive to our hunches and our stomach butterflies, and to understanding that we are all connected and the Earth is much more than just the ground on which we build our homes. Mother Earth is Nature, and Nature is us all.

I don't condemn meat eating, nor will I label it as wrong. We are all different and each body requires different types of fuel. I have met beautiful people with the same intentions of doing good that do eat meat, however, they agree with me on sourcing food responsibly, buying organic and local food when possible, ditching processed foods, and eating what you can understand and can pronounce. Lastly, I have two requests: try practicing #MeatlessMondays, and do an act of love for yourself, cook!

Chef

"Anyone can cook, but only the fearless can be great."

– Chef Auguste Gusteau, Ratatouille

The restaurant industry is a fearsome place. Restaurant critics are maniacs with power demanding perfection. A food critique can make your restaurant shine, or can demolish your dreams like a crumbling pie. Traditional cooking is modeled after French cuisine, with its mother sauces, heavy creams, pastries, *gastriques.* In a way, cooking is a very classical and traditional art. Most chefs hit the wall of criticism before finding success and find that their innovative ways of making food are rejected. But most of those who stick to what they do perform one single undeniable act: they follow their gut. Those who stick to their passion, roots, and culture can succeed and create dishes that bring them success on their own terms, like Chef Francis Mallman of Argentina, or Chef Alex Atala of Brazil. Those who take a machete to the protocol and dare to serve outside the plating guidelines may find true style and meaning in their food, like Chef Massimo Bottura of Italy, or Chef Grant Achatz of Chicago. Those with a sense of purpose in creating food find an unstoppable melody in their art, like Matthew Kenney.

Matthew Kenney is one of those chefs who risked it all on a shift to plant-based cuisine. Having spent years as an established French-trained celebrity chef in New York opening restaurants and writing books on the art of traditional cuisine, he decided to make a change and succeed again with a new type of cuisine. He is responsible for making "vegan" a culinary term rather than just an ethical connotation. He has built an empire around plant-based cuisine that has given it the reputation and respect that any other type of cuisine enjoys. Now, he has high-end completely raw plant-based restaurants in Maine, Los Angeles, and Miami that have been reviewed as the best of the best. He has also opened academies both online and on-site to continue his mission to craft the future of food with quality ingredients and the most sophisticated and elevated cuisine techniques.

I had the fortune to train at his academy, to work with his team, and to meet him personally. His approach to cuisine is so detailed and precise that every drop of water matters, every stroke on the plate matters, and every slice of the knife adds to the eating experience. After completing several of his courses, gathering my fundamental cooking skills, and finally being mentored by a professional who respected the act of cooking and eating as much as I did, I transitioned from just a home cook to a plant-based food artist. Now, I dance to his tune, making a full-time career out of what was once only simple curiosity.

Big changes are happening in our industry. Every day you see more vegan options on menus, more plant-based festivals, fairs, and more completely vegan restaurants popping up. In February of 2016, well-known restaurateur Ravi DeRossi decided to turn his 15 meat-based restaurants in New York into vegan eateries inspired by Polynesian cuisine. He stated, "I'm more worried about my conscience and living without the weight on my shoulder of the damage I'm doing, and the suffering of animals."[*]

You see, there's cooking for survival, and then there's cooking for art. Plant-based cuisine merges these two. When you choose to cook or eat in a plant-based, you are voting for better quality of life. Plant-based cooking is political, it is social, and it's real. Whether your plate looks like a Pollock picture or is simply a bouquet of cauliflower, I assure you that you can find beauty in it, because your reasons for choosing plant-based food will always be inspired by being better.

---

[*]   http://vegnews.com/articles/page.do?pageId=7481&catId=1

Nourishing Path

- Do you crave any foods in particular?
- Are you going through any emotional situations that interfere with your work, relationships, or health?
- What activity do you use to relax your mind? Can you find any type of movement or practice to bring more joy and relaxation into your life?
- Can you think of any situation in which you had to make a choice and you trusted your gut instinct? What was the outcome of that?
- In what kinds of intelligence do you excel?
- Is your job or routine in alignment with your purpose?
- Are you willing to demand better quality foods for you and your loved ones?
- Are you willing to take responsibility for your health?

Nourishing Tips

- Take a cooking class
- Order from services such as Blue Apron or Green Chef to inspire you to cook at home and share the experience with your family
- Avoid any "diet" products or synthetic sugars
- Join the worldwide #meatlessmonday movement and avoid eating meat on Mondays
- Go to a plant based restaurant out of curiosity and enjoy the experience

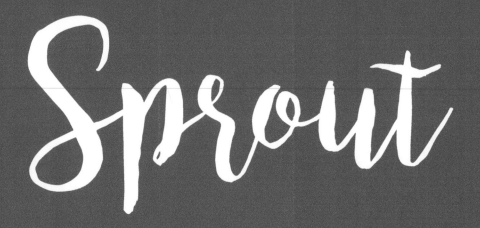

"The future will belong to the Naturesmart --those individuals, families, businesses, and political leaders who develop a deeper understanding of the transformative power of the natural world and who balance the virtual with the real. The more high-tech we become, the more Nature we need."

— Richard Louv

Kale

"I love myself, the most quietest, simplest, most powerful revolution ever."

- Nayyirah Waheed

I remember having vivid conversations about obesity with different friends which stuck with me for a lifetime. One was ages before I even knew that kale existed. I was talking with an older friend of mine, although we were both still in our teens. We were chatting about things we couldn't stand, and he brought up fat people. He went off about it, trying to understand why people would allow themselves get into that situation; he blamed them and condemned them. I just stared at him, unaware that he was introducing a new concept into my subconscious. Another memorable talk about this subject was just in the last couple years, however, I had not yet become aware of the psychological power of food, as I was very new indeed to the power of healthy foods and a healthy lifestyle. This friend of mine had a very restrictive way of seeing food; for her, food was just fuel, and that's where it ended. She was commenting on another friend of mine who worked in the health industry. My girlfriend just couldn't understand how someone who worked for the health department could be obese. This time, I became very angry at her, since I knew the friend she was criticizing and thought nothing of him but that he was a kindred soul. What I overlooked, however, was that by trying to defend my friend, I too was judging "fatness", as if being fat was something "bad" that had happened to him.

"Obesity" is not something that is just happening to you or me, it's a *global* crisis that is manifesting on an individual level. "Fat" on the other hand or "gaining weight" is only a personal symptom connected to our emotional turmoil.

Sadly, this is the way we blame ourselves as well. This is why we punish ourselves for gaining weight or being called fat. We restrict ourselves with food, or even worse, we force ourselves to exhausting efforts at the gym with self-loathing thoughts as the motivation. We live in an era that promotes superficiality. Focusing on the body to judge the soul is a sign of insecurity, pain, fear, and of having been robbed of our basic core value: to love and be loved.

How easy would it be if 1+1=2 in every scenario. But it does not; you can't just apply logic, math, or science to understand our neuroses. Those are tools, but do not lead to the only truth. If it was that easy, we would all eat the same food for breakfast, lunch, and dinner, dress the same way, have the same job, and weigh exactly the same. We are all equal, but we are not the same. We are emotional beings. Food affects us all in different ways, however, what rules our metabolism is not how many kale smoothies we are drinking or how many calories we are burning, but how we are feeling emotionally, spiritually, and physically.

Eating is an act of the mind, body and soul. You are fed throughout your life by your own thoughts, by people's conversations, by your love and your fear. Being obese has nothing to do with a 'will power problem' – and I hope my friend from back in the day comes across this insight – being obese is a symptom of the soul screaming to be addressed. Gaining weight is an accumulation of energy being stored in our bodies because we don't want to use it yet. Perhaps this is because we don't want to speak up; we may have a wounding truth we are afraid to share, like having been sexually abused or having experienced a traumatic event, and now we use our bodies as a protective shield or hidden wall. We may gain weight because we are stressed, because we can't forgive, or can't make enough money. We may gain weight because we are cheating ourselves out of our own personal power, what we came to this earth to do. We may gain weight when we are in fear or when we don't want to let go. Collectively, we are gaining weight as the "wake up call for a life out of balance asking us to rethink our relationship with the earth, [and] with our industrialized doings"*. We are gaining weight on a global scale due to our Machiavellian obsession with greed.

Physiologically speaking, every angst feeling we experience is described as a stressor on the body. Stress throws our bodies out of balance by invoking the sympathetic nervous system response and unleashing a set of hormones meant to protect us. One of its main roles when stressed is to store fat as a survival mechanism. When we are in constant stress, our adrenal glands try to cover it up by pumping more adrenaline and cortisol, eventually exhausting energy reserves and ending up with adrenal fatigue. Then, when one gland is out of whack, it pulls on another gland, eventually from another organ or physical system, potentially from the lymphatic, cardiovascular, digestive, or endocrine systems, and our whole body falls into dis-ease. All chronic dis-eases, cancers, hormone unbalances, headaches, and digestive disturbances date back to a thought, a feeling, or a hurtful emotion you've lived through.

When we are in such a state, we can't keep pumping kale smoothies into ourselves and working ourselves to death in the gym without first uncovering what is really happening to us. Your body would appreciate more healthy foods coming in, but first, it wants your love.

All of us are walking the streets of these cities with some kind of discomfort. The discomfort can be temporary or permanent. You can choose to numb the pain with pills, diets, alcohol, or restrictions. But body minus food doesn't equal weight loss, unlocking what's holding your spirit back is the magic wand, the helping hand that could bring you closer to your destiny. After losing weight, 99% of people on a weight loss diet gain it back. It's not that

---

* The Slow Down Diet, Marc David pg. 167

they didn't continue following their diet or that they lack will power, they just worked on the surface, addressing weight gain with nothing but left brain thinking and purposeful arithmetic. However, that 1% found a deeper reason to wake up in the morning other than trying to fit in their skinny jeans. That 1% changed their perspective; they are inspired to live, to make things happen, and to accept themselves as they are.

Who's to say you should weigh less or more? After various studies, science hasn't been able to unanimously determine if gaining weight is a sign of disease or health. We are all unique! We are not molded after anyone but ourselves. There's no return slip to our momma's belly because we are too skinny or too tall. Gaining weight is a sign that there is a need to address something greater. In some cases it can be a good thing.

Our world needs a paradigm shift. What we are being fed everyday through the media, in the average TV show, and on social media is polluting our minds. We are being brainwashed to think we must achieve perfection of the body, when what should be promoted instead is the cultivation of our values, our self-love, and our growth as a community, respecting and taking care of our only planetary home.

It tears at my heart when I hear my grandma saying she won't have another cookie because she will get fat. How on earth have we come to such an extreme, when a 90+ year old beautiful woman weighing less than 110 pounds fears being called fat?! I feel responsible, as part of this generation, for her innocent sense of guilt, and so I want to make things right.

Join me.

Let's obsess about things that matter than can create a positive change, let's be extreme in our ways so even our elders feel the need to change no matter how late they think it is. It's never too late. If you can live your last years in joy and love and with much more gumption, why wouldn't you?

If we can start now, why don't we?

It's the hurtful thoughts, the stressed life with no time for personal enjoyment, the junk food and other life-lacking foods, the synthetic sugars, the lab-created foods, and the lack of responsibility for our own health that hurt our spirits. It's seeing ourselves as material objects rather than powerful souls that is hurting our collective capacity to love.

Kudos to my kind friend for working in the health industry. We often teach what we need to learn. After all, our own suffering is the best teacher we can have to give us insight into the suffering of others. To heal our own pain can be the motivation needed to serve others.

By all means get your morning started with a kale smoothie, but ask yourself first, is the reason you want to change your habits born out of love or fear?

Plate

We are sitting at the table to eat, already feeling exhausted. We subconsciously think food is our enemy, and so shoveling food into our mouths is just one more thing we have to do. There are people who prefer to turn the TV on to eat; with a mechanically rotating motion, they stick the spoonful of cereal into their mouth, then back to the bowl to scoop some more, and repeat. Or maybe the one that we see most often in our current environments, people who eat while staring at a monitor, talking on a cell phone at the same time. Or perhaps you snack at every time you see food, and stuff your mouth with candy bars, feeling hungry even though you ate only 15 minutes ago. Whether you are numbing yourself to eat because you don't like food, are afraid to eat, can't stop eating, or are too busy to set aside twenty minutes to take in your meal, these actions are not something you are doing to food, these are behaviors that are express through food the relationship you have with yourself.

Not taking the time to eat while you work is as if to say that your work is more important than you, or you are not important enough in your own life to dedicate twenty minutes of lunch to yourself. It's ironic, because what happens down the line is that when you get sick you can't show up for work, and you can't show up for yourself. In this case, sickness is necessary to ground you and to hopefully open your eyes to your responsibility for your own health.

Eating is as connected to nourishing yourself as it is to selecting quality ingredients. Your job of nourishing your body doesn't stop at having a healthy meal prep service drop the food off at your doorstep.

Food that comes into your mouth becomes part of you. Tell me what you eat, and I'll tell you what you are made of, right? But for the food to address its purpose, it needs to be received *by you*.

Digestion doesn't start in the stomach. The digestive process starts once you've decided to eat and sit down at the table. It's what is known as the *Cephalic Digestive Phase*. Think of an example from yoga practice: when you arrive on your mat and the class is about to begin, you don't just jump right into ekam pose, the teacher actually leads a quick breathing exercise, or salutes with an OM or meditation practice to get you ready for your postures. You need to prepare your mind, get rid of the traffic jam-stress, the thoughts about the papers you have to sign at work, and simply surrender yourself to the practice. The meditation before the practice is what the Cephalic Phase is to eating. It's an invitation to the mind to land here.

It's the preparation stage, the flirting before dating. Then yoga; the practice of stretching your body and working with your body is what nourishment it's all about, it's that relationship between you and your [eating] practice.

The Cephalic phase is turned on by the smells coming from the kitchen, by the beautiful plate of food served by your loved one, by the view out the window, by the music and the ambience, even by the good company sharing the meal with you. Enter your favorite bakery, and as soon you walk past the door, your mind has already started imagining the different flavors and textures you are about to enjoy. You have already begun to salivate.

Cephalic means "of the head", so indeed, it is waking up the head brain in order to alert the other organs and second brain about your date with your plate. In his book *The Slow Down Diet*, Marc David states how digestive power and caloric burning capacity is turned up to 80% when we respect this head-phase. That means your ability to break down food, to absorb nutrients, and to know when to stop eating is related to paying attention when you start eating.

An exercise I like to do with my daughter is to give thanks for our food before we eat. Sometimes she's into what I serve, other times I have to grab her attention to make her eat. Whatever the case, in order to focus her into our eating experience, we recite, *"Gracias Madre por la Comida tan Rica,"* which translates, "Thank you Mother for the delicious food." We both hold our plate up as if we are about to cheer and set the start of our eating practice. When I'm alone, I recite in my head, "Thank you Mother Earth for nourishing me with your love and wisdom." Also, when I'm about to cook for my clients or for myself, I look at my note board in my kitchen and read, "Thank you Plant Mother for nourishing these foods," as a way of blessing the food and offering my best intentions for the meal. Giving thanks for your food or saying a prayer before you eat aligns your body and soul into the moment; it prepares your mind and your entire digestive system to receive what you are feeding it. A simple "Thanks" will always do, or try thanking the person that cooked for you. Alternatively, sharing the common "Bon Appetit!" with your co-workers or friends can start you and your friends on your way to proper digestion.

Full digestive power also has to do with our great friend *breathing*! It's actually our *panacea*. There is nothing in this life you can do without breathing, and every single thing you do can improve when you improve the quality of your breathing. Some studies have shown that when you breathe four repetitive counts inand then four repetitive counts out, you can put your body in detoxification mode. Or if you practice a 1-minute meditation called "Ujjayi" taught by Ayurveda medicine, which consists on breathing deeply in and out through your nose for 30 seconds and then sitting still for 30 more seconds, you can bring your body into a state of relaxation. In contrast, shallow breathing actually turns on the stress response[*]. If you think about a situation when you experienced panic, you can recall how quick and short your breaths were. Shallow breathing is associated with anxiety and nervousness. When you exercise, if you have no control of your breathing you can deplete your body to the point of exhaustion, and can actually gain weight. However, if you keep a deep in/out nose breathing rhythm, magical things can happen, like burning more calories. Slow deep breathing from my abdomen is what I held onto when I gave birth – it was my natural anesthetic. Controlling your breath calms your body and emotions and can also help you deepen your sleep, reduce insomnia, help develop your intuition and assist you with making better choices[**].

---

[*]   The 3-Season Diet, John Douillard, pg. 5
[**]   Deepak Chopra – Sleep Meditation, YouTube Video, min. 00:45 – https://www.youtube.com/watch?v=ixscQ3t1oJY

If before eating you take three to five deep breaths, you are automatically turning up that calorie-burning fire within, and I can assure you, as you make this practice a nourishing habit, your digestion will improve dramatically.

I find it very interesting that the norm is to ask about how many calories are in a food without any knowledge whatsoever of what a calorie is. A calorie is a measurement unit that determines how much heat is released from an object when burned. That object can either be edible, or made of plastic, wood, chemicals, etc. Anything can have calories! The number of calories listed on the back of the package of the foods is completely irrelevant to the masses, because all of our capacity to burn calories is individual and is determined by how much oxygen there is in each of our stomachs, which is pumped down there by slow deep abdominal breathing. You already know that for fire to exist it needs oxygen. The same concept applies here. If there's oxygen in the stomach, if I'm breathing deeply and I'm relaxed when eating, then my calorie-burning capacity is fired up.

The amount of oxygen in my stomach is completely different from yours. It could be true to say that I can digest an apple much quickly than you, but also that I can digest an apple today effortlessly because I'm happy and relaxed; but tomorrow if I'm stressed and tense, I would probably get a stomach ache afterwards and wouldn't be able to tolerate the fruit at all. So those 95 calories from an apple can turn into 950 on a bad day.

We cannot measure our success with numbers any more, not in any realm. The amount of money you have means nothing if you are depressed and sad. The quality of life comes from the emotions, the ability to accept joy, the embodiment of our own stories, and the ability to be present here, today, celebrating the now.

Looking back at our nutrition timeline since the 1950s, when we first became collectively conscious about our weight, the message sold to us through the media about our bodies was to "lose weight to achieve happiness;" then it transitioned to "eat that because it's healthy," which then will make you skinny and then happy. I suggest we call off the hunt and call living by its name; *be happy!* Which means you are already healthy, because you make the right conscious decisions for you and your loved ones, which also translates to loving yourself!

Some people stick to numbers because they want to control and measure progress and because they like logics and straightforward answers. That's left brain thinking, that's our masculine side talking for us. That's okay sometimes, but just as science is not the absolute truth, to limit ourselves only to what we can see vs. what we can feel is to live in disharmony with our own nature.

When you ask about calories, you are in fear of those toxic nutritional beliefs I have so passionately raved about: "food is the enemy," "food makes me fat," "fat is bad." In truth you just need to see yourself with different eyes, the eyes of love, and demand *real quality* food. Food that grows in the darkness and sprouts in silence from the dirt. Food that we pull from the body of Mother Earth. Food that is nourished with her love and wisdom.

Who cares how much you weigh?! You are simply some number of pounds of beating-heart, sensual-pure organic matter called Nature.

Make the right question about food: where does it come from? Take deep breaths before you grab your fork, give thanks for your meal, and fall in love with the practice of eating!

Sun

We owe our entire continuum of existence to one star, the sun. Without the sun, water wouldn't evaporate to form clouds, which then sprinkle our lands to moisten the earth and sprout seeds. Without the sun, trees and plants couldn't exist; there would be no light to photosynthesize, no oxygen to breathe. Without the sun there would be no darkness, because we wouldn't be able to recognize what light is. No sun, no sunflowers. No sun, no vitamin D.

There's an unspoken order in Nature that keeps its essence wild. It is a structure, so to speak, to be respected and honored by all its living beings. We often think of "wild" as chaotic or unstructured, but although there are no straight lines in Nature, you can find perfect mathematical patterns of growth and shapes in its entire kingdom from the growth pattern of a snail shell, to the perfect formation of hexagonal wall cells on a bee's hive. Chaos in Nature is rare. Our planet revolves as it orbits around its king, the sun, 365 times a year, keeping the cycle of Nature flawless, with all its springs, hurricanes, volcanoes, streams and sunsets.

Since our bodies are part of that animal kingdom and part of the perfection of Nature, they also respond to the sun when they properly function. We have an internal clock that is stimulated by light, a 24-hour cycle called the Circadian Rhythm. The Circadian Rhythm is the structure on which we ought to rely to live our everyday lives. It tells us when to wake up and when to go to sleep, what time to eat, what time to rest and relax, and what time to have sex. However, technology is moving so fast that we cannot keep up with the changes that are being thrown at us. I guess we are just part of the experimental process, but I trust that we will be able to harmonize our never-ending energy for creation with having a synergetic connection with Nature.

Our Circadian Rhythm is dependent on the sun. Our bodies wake up at sunrise; even though you may not notice it, instinctively you will stretch, flutter your eyes, or wake up and then go back to sleep around this time. This is the first signal of a new start. That means that our digestive system is also getting the wake-up call, and so the rest of your systems are too. By noon, when the sun is at its zenith, our digestive fire and our energies are turned up. This is the time when we should be having our biggest meal of the day, because our digestive system is wide awake, and it's expecting food to work with to provide us with energy for the rest of the day. Lunch should be anytime from noon to three p.m. After this time, as the sun "moves" to the west, our bodies start cooling down into a more calming energy.

Food should most often be eaten with the presence of the sun, meaning, our last dinner of the day (or "supper", which comes from the French "soup" for "light dinner") should be eaten right before sunset, when our digestive system is performing its last run. After sunset, a couple of things happen; the red shadows and rays from the sun stimulate our pineal gland into relaxation mode, taking the body into sleep/rest time. Candlesand fire were used in the past, which mimics the color and warmth properties of the sun to keep us close to each other, more quiet and intimate, preparing our entire organism to rest, sleep and detox.

Yet, as time progresses, rest, sleep, detox, and intimacy are the last thing we are experiencing in our bedrooms. According to the New York Times, "about sixty percent of the U.S. population is struggling with sleep at least a few times each week."[*] One of the root causes of this problem is due to our misuse of technology. The blue light emitted by all the monitor screens we look at, including our smart phones and tablets, confuses our pineal gland, which is responsible for the release of our bodies' sleep hormone, melatonin. The blue light mimics the sunlight we should be receiving between sunrise and sunset, not at bed time – light stimulation right before we go to bed causes confusion to our circadian rhythms, resulting in interrupted sleep.

Do not underestimate the power of sleep. Just as you look at diet as a tool to reach health, there are few things about your lifestyle that you can tweak to help you maintain nirvana as your everyday state. While you sleep, your body goes into detox mode. Your brain enters into the most important process of its existence, that of rebuilding itself, restoring tissue, and balancing the rest of your nervous system. During your sleep you hit the refresh button to revive your creativity, vitality, intelligence and overall development – this is the reason why kids sleep so much. The younger they are the more time they spend napping, resting, and growing.

A good night of 7-8 hours of sleep is generally what we need. Some folks can run on only four hours, but to reach such a state, your lifestyle must support the vitality and vibrancy of your health so that you require only a few hours of recovery each night. It's possible, but not for stressed, overworked, sad, or angry people. Sleep helps regulate your hormones, and indeed hormones are a main reason why so many of us are out of whack.

We are fighting our own Nature; it's just that we don't know what we are doing. I'm sure none of us spend hours scrolling down Facebook in bed with the intention of killing our body's melatonin and throwing the hypothalamus out of synch, but doing so is messing up with our sleep. We must reevaluate our lives and reject mediocrity. We were meant to live at our full spectrum, and if something isn't right, dig deeper and you'll find what's in your way. You will find solutions to your problems.

For example, you can download an app for your computer called *f.lux* that will synch your computer's clock with sunrise and sunset in your area and dim the screen brightness after sunset automatically. Or if you have an iPhone or iPad, Apple also came up with the solution of offering an option like the app mentioned above to dim your screen after sunset. You can also

---

[*] Sara Gottfried http://live.well.org/wp-content/uploads/2015/09/Module-5-Sleep-Transcript.pdf

get a pair of good ol' BluBlockers sunglasses and wear them while working or playing on your device. However, my intention is not so much to tell you how to hack the system, but how to become more nourished from the inside out to really reach your health and happiness and anchor it to your forever present. Doesn't gathering around the fire to tell stories and cuddle next to your loved ones sound like the right thing to do before going to bed? Maybe we can use some of our ancestral wisdom to make us more human beings, and less human machines. What if your bedroom became your sanctuary and you honored that space by bringing in elements that added to your tranquility instead of robbing you of your melatonin? Did you know that your sleeping brainwave patterns operate at 1 to 3 hertz per second? The average light bulb runs at 60 hertz!* Leave all electronics outside your bedroom door and get a small light box, a couple of candles, or a red light bulb in your room if you need the light, and simply prepare this space to be the one where you surrender to sleep and dream, or as Pedram Shojai says, designate your bedroom only for sleeping and making love.

I find the perfection of Nature simply astonishing and humbling. It is said that everything we need is to be found within a 100 foot radius. The sun is always there – nearly 93 million miles away, yet its splendor and warmth are able to caress our skin as soon as we step out the door. The sun also provides us with one of the vitamins that our health depends on, vitamin D. If you thought milk was the main source of vitamin D, you are not that far from the truth, because dairy milk comes from pasture-fed animals, which if properly raised should be turned out to pasture during the spring, when they are exposed to the sun's radiance as well as the healthiest stage of the growing grass, which also provides vitamin D. Hence, high quality cheese and milk should come from spring pasture-raised ruminants.

I'm not opposed to having butter, or ghee, (which is clarified butter lacking casein, a protein that is harmful to some people.) I can't have dairy, but if my family is having it I always stress to them the need to get the best quality possible. If you are buying commercial grade butter from factory farm cows, chances are there are no natural vitamins in these products, and if the products are advertised as providing these nutrients, they were synthetically fortified. Since the animals spend their lives in steel cages under a shaded roof and are fed grains including soy and corn which do not belong in their diet, it's impossible for cows or chickens to provide through their milk or eggs the essential nutrients we look for in these foods.

Raw dairy is a great source of nutrients, vitamins, and healthy bacteria. Although is not legally sold at regular stores for human consumption, you can find it at farmers markets sold as "pet food" – although every states has different rules. This of course is not part of a vegan regimen, but I'm not about being dogmatic and religious; my lifestyle and suggestions are about being in harmony with our habitat. Raw dairy products often come from local farmers who raise their animals in a natural and safe environment, promoting life and respect for living systems. I support their regenerative agriculture and ethics, so I have raw dairy on occasion, as more of a delicacy than a staple item. Raw dairy can be better assimilated and digested than its homogenized and pasteurized counterpart, even for those with lactose intolerance or dairy sensitivities.

---

*   The Urban Monk, Pedram Shojai pg. 75, 76

Dairy makes of a great carrier for vitamin D because it also contains fat. Vitamin D is fat-soluble. Our skin is coated with a thin invisible layer of fat whose sole purpose is to absorb sunlight to convert into vitamin D. Insufficient omega-3s or healthy fat in our diet can cause a vitamin D deficiency.

Vitamin D is essential for a million functions in our bodies; it regulates our mood and energy, prevents depression, and most importantly, it helps us absorb and assimilate calcium. Here is another misconception about dairy: it's not milk that makes our bones strong, it's actually the combination of vitamin D, calcium, collagen and fat. Actually, there's so much calcium in milk that there can be an overdose of this mineral in our system. If we lack vitamin D, this calcium then finds its way to our joints or other parts of our body and is accumulated as deposits, or our body starts leeching minerals from our blood in order to assimilate the large quantities of calcium, which can resulting in depletion of other minerals, and even osteoporosis.

Too much calcium is what leads to osteoporosis since it makes our bones brittle. To counteract the overdose, we need collagen, enough vitamin D, and more anti-inflammatory healthy fats.

When we lack Vitamin D, it can wreak havoc on our entire system, including our endocrine system. Solution: get in the habit of taking a short 10 minute walk around your neighborhood in the morning, maybe even at sunrise, or else at work after lunch. When spending time in the sun, don't put on sunscreen, as this will block the sun's nourishment of your skin, just be cautious of your exposure time. As you walk around the block, or the park or beach, breathe deeply, which will instantly relax you – now you have enriched your day by practicing life-nourishing techniques that have always been available to you.

Surprisingly, Vitamin D is one of the vitamins our population is most deficient in. Ironic, since we can just step out into the sun for 10 minutes to naturally get what we need to fully thrive.

...The solutions are at of our fingertips!

Blood

> "It turns out good health looks more like a
> partnership with Nature."
>
> *– Pedram Shojai*

Pleasure, sex, and even eating are all natural human habits seen as taboos in our culture. We have a tendency to feel guilty about our most natural functions, such as excreting substances, sweating, smelling, having an appetite, or going through our moon cycle. Some of these natural expressions of our bodies may not be pleasant for some, but they shouldn't make one ashamed. It's built into our genetics and biology; it's what makes us living beings and part of expanding evolution.

The way we are disassociated from our Nature just makes us even more confused about our instincts and collective intuition. For instance, scent can be its own language, by which we signal potential mates of our reproduction phase. Some of us find our partner's smell so attractive, while their close relatives can't stand it – which tends to prevent mating within the biological family. Yet our response as a society to all the smells, fluids, and natural results of our biology is to hide them, to condemn them, to eliminate them, or to numb them. Nowadays, there's a cream, a soap bar, or a pill to conceal our biology. When we become a society dependent on synthetic products for our daily existence, we cannot fully thrive to our maximum potential. We become so desensitized to our own Nature that we become desensitized to Nature itself. Our bodies become vessels for toxic chemicals that pollute our pores, our cells, and our minds. We lose our sense of smell by filling up our noses with synthetic air fresheners, which prevent us from stopping and truly smelling the roses. We wash our hands with antibacterial soaps, killing 99.9% of our own bacteria, which also kills the good bacteria that protect us and keep our systems in balance, resulting in all sorts of new allergies and frequent colds. We apply synthetic-based, aluminum-containing products to our armpits to eliminate odors, making us prone to more chronic illnesses, thyroid imbalances and even cancers. Why can't we stop for a second and ask instead what could be causing an unpleasant smell? Terrible body odor is usually associated with toxins and metal toxicity caused by a poor diet.

The more we evolve, the more we are enslaving ourselves to the pharmacy aisles instead of increasing our freedom. We have even found ways to hack the feminine reproductive system by disrupting our hormones to prevent pregnancy, overlooking the multitude of "side effects such blinding methods as the use of birth control pills are causing in us. Women who use synthetic contraceptives are becoming more estrogen predominant, which is a leading cause of breast cancer, ovarian cancer, and liver cancer. Birth control pills increase the risk of blood clots and strokes; they also cause imbalances in our immune systems and changes in our natural flora, making our bodies prone to infections due to yeast and other pathogenic bacteria[*] – and yet we ask why women are not fertile anymore?!

We are the only living species having problems procreating, whether due to male or female infertility. This is not a matter of going to the doctor and asking, "what's wrong with me?" Better to ask, WHAT'S WRONG WITH US? The inability of a species to reproduce means the end of that species.

It's about time we start asking ourselves the right questions and start to look at our problems from a collective perspective. Carl Jung speaks of the collective unconscious as the deep common unconscious thinking that we share. It's time we start to collectively transform our feelings of fear, guilt, and shame into understanding that we are all part of Nature. The plant world offers all the answers; it offers us a sense of belonging that when truly experienced, can help us feel how beautiful life is and how necessary it is for us to align with the Earth. That's how you spell freedom.

I know asking you to change your lifelong brands for flower essences or coconut oil may seem overwhelming, but there's no need to be so drastic right away. Begin to make the transition for yourself in ways that feel comfortable, and who knows, maybe you'll discover a new hobby of mixing cooking ingredients into soap pastes. My bathrooms pretty much looks like an extension of my kitchen, and that happened over time. Next to my toothbrush you can find coconut oil and apple cider vinegar; next to my bathtub there are mineral salts, Dr. Bronner's liquid soaps, and essential oils. Over the years I have come to understand that food is not limited to what we can eat, but to anything that can be absorbed by our five senses. Our skin is our biggest organ, and everything we apply to it is absorbed with much more intense effects than if eaten. Simply changing your mainstream detergent-containing soap for an eco-friendly soap is a good way to start. Visiting a health food store to buy your toothpaste can be a painless transition step. Everyone moves at their own pace. Wherever you are in your path, make small modifications that can bring you joy, new outlooks and new experiences.

Pleasure, sex, and eating shouldn't be forbidden but honored. It's in our constitution to seek pleasure and avoid pain. Pleasure relaxes us; it turns on our parasympathetic nervous system response, which is the switch in our organism that accounts for perfect function of our bodies; total burning capacity, metabolic rate, digestive fire, and full nutrient assimilation and absorption. When we eat we are receiving pleasure from our food, from our companions sitting at the table with us, and from the nourishing moment

---

[*]   Hashimoto's Thyroiditis, Izabella Wentz, pg. 207

itself. However, when we are stressed, afraid of eating, or in resistance to eating, we signal cortisol to take over our system for protection; and then in that prolonged state of stress, we live in fear, anxiety, and sickness. Cortisol is a primordial hormone that when properly working helps with the functioning of a number of different activities in our bodies. But when it is in dysfunction, it can disrupt our sleep and tranquility, absorption of nutrients, insulin regulation, weight retention, and even our emotions. When we avoid pleasure and prevent ourselves from experiencing life to the fullest,then cortisol is forced to take over and the "beauty" of this hormone turns to a "beast". Joe Cross put it best: *we become fat, sick and nearly dead.*

Biologically speaking, pleasure is part of our genetic coding to enjoy the acts of eating and of sex, which are two of the most fundamentally important activities for the continuation of humankind. If we don't eat, we don't grow. If we don't get the nutrients we need, we can't function properly. If we don't nourish our bodies with quality foods and activities, we get sick. The act of eating [and sex] is rewarded by pleasure itself! Even if you find yourself starving in the middle of the day with only a few minutes to eat, enjoy them by using visualization and the capabilities of your mind to give your body the nourishing energy it needs to continue serving you during your harsh, fast-paced, stressful day.

Sex, sexual energy, sexual beings: all of us are sexual beings. Everything that we look at was created by the merging of two energies, idea and action, female and male, flower and butterfly. However, sex in our culture is the most misunderstood, judged, and punished desire. In actuality, the way you eat is directly reflected in the way you have sex. Because the understanding that you have of your body, the respect you give it, and the way you nourish it are all represented in the way that you play with your body, the way that you seek sensuality, and in the way you relate with your partner. Whatever touches, caresses, and love you receive and share with your partner are the same energy you give yourself. Such thinking is the same one you are going to bring to the table when nourishing your body.

When you respect yourself as a human being, you are contributing to the collective thinking of our world. We are tapping into that realm and changing our memes to demand a better life, better values, and more love for our entire universe.

How about celebrating the entry of a girl into womanhood at her first menstruation like a once in a lifetime experience? What if we honored our menstrual cycle instead of tolerating it?

When those days come we seldom celebrate them, unless of course our period's arrival means no unforeseen pregnancy, even though the blood that spills from between our legs means so much more than a sigh after a wild night with no condom at hand. That blood means life. It grants women the wonderful gift of creating a precious soul.

Every ejaculation, every orgasm, every sweat, every breath, and every blood cycle are a reminder that there is life and creative energy all around us.

Connecting with that creative sacred energy can only bring us more joy and more understanding. Instead of hypnotizing our hormones with "the pill", there is a natural way of better understand our transformations. It's called the natural "Fertility Awareness Method". It's a system that teaches you how to read your body signals and your temperature so you can know with certainty when you are ovulating or when you should have sex with your partner, either to become pregnant or to naturally avoid pregnancy. The FAM teaches us how to be in harmony with our circadian rhythm, and it illuminates our female energetic dependency on the moon.

It's no coincidence we call it our "moon cycle", since it's the lunar [light] pattern that triggers our ovulation. Before the presence of artificial light at night, women were more in synch with the moon, starting the reproductive cycle with each new moon, then ovulating 12–14 days later when the moon was at its fullest, which meant less melatonin production (since there's more moonlight at the full moon) and more ovulation power[*].

Living in a more natural way cannot guarantee a disease-free life, because we are all vulnerable to stress. However, the recovery speed of someone who has treated his or her body with respect is light-years ahead of everyone else. The more aligned you are with your own nature, your natural environment, your food, your spiritual practices, your relationships, and your work, the more likely you are to rapidly return to health and happiness. The more toxins swimming in your blood, the more insensitive you'll be of natural remedies, and holistic methods. There's a built-up resistance we have sometimes towards a more natural path. But as a wise person once told me, the more resistance we have to something, the more we need it.

There are studies that prove depression can be cured by spending time in Nature, by changing your posture, or by simply smiling more. Stress can be reduced by taking a walk in the park in the sun, going for a swim in the ocean, or playing in the sand. Ayurvedic and Chinese medicine are systems of healing that have studied the human body and our connection with Nature for thousands of years. They propose healing our bodies with herbs, a balanced diet, and mindful practices. All these methods have something in common, it's called "grounding" or as explained in recent studies, "earthing". Clint Ober, scientist and inventor of grounding technology, concludes, "hormonal fluctuations within the metabolism are referenced to innate rhythms that electromagnetically emanate from the Earth itself[**]. Meaning, when we are out of synch with the earth's "palpitations" we are literally unsettled. Psychologically we are floating, lost, and confused; physiologically speaking we are uneased, and our hormones are all over the place.

The Merriam-Webster definition of a grounded person is "a person who is sensible and has a good understanding of what is really important in life"[***]. By grounding ourselves with Nature, we can accomplish the order and alignment of our body and soul. Grounding is to simply spend time in Nature, to connect to the source, to charge our batteries with the mother energy of the earth; these can be accomplished by swimming in natural bodies of water, dipping your feet under the sand, getting some sunlight, doing some gardening, laying on the grass, climbing trees, spending more time outdoors.

---

[*]   Your Fertility Signals, Merryl Winstein, pg. 85
[**]   Longevity Now, David Wolfe, pg. 199
[***]   http://www.merriam-webster.com/dictionary/grounded

Harmony

A couple weeks ago I attended a vegan festival near Miami. Although you wouldn't expect it, I felt skeptical about going because nowadays I often avoid groups or meetups on *veganism*. I have a problem defining myself as a *vegan* as well. Granted, the extreme mentality of wanting to eradicate all conformity, creating new social standards for what is right to eat or not eat, and simply detaching myself from the indirect violence I was creating with my poor food choices was necessary. Yet as I look back, I see my becoming *vegan* as a cleansing phase. It was a necessary phase so I could "clean house" and get rid of the garbage thoughts that stood in my way; it was taking the veil off my eyes and reclaiming my power over my health. Veganism has a beautiful resonance with our world; it promotes kindness, awareness, train of thoughts that are much needed in our hurried lives. It gives our rebellion a sense of direction and purpose, towards creation and not destruction.

However, as time progresses and I delve deeper into studies on the psychology of food, and by simply noticing how change and trends work in our society, I've came to see how being part of fill-in-the-blank diet is blinding us to the fundamental reason to why we chose to become vegan, or paleo, or raw or whatever it is in the first place.

We are replacing our religion with a diet. We think if we have a piece of cheese or bread we are bad people! I was recently tagged to a Facebook post on *veganism* asking people to pledge not to sit next to anyone that eats meat! I find this behavior offensive; I find it disempowering and fanatical.

Back at the festival, as soon as I walked through the door, I heard a woman on the stage giving a talk on how vegans should not allow themselves to be called "plant-based". She continued her argument by saying that plant-based limits itself only to food, and thus this "diet" does not save monkeys in cages in Africa if a person wears leather, for example. I looked around, gently took hold of my daughter, found the exit and left. The point here is not how many animals we are saving, the bottom line is to get to the root causes and seed more kindness and love in all of us immediately. It is disconnection with others and with our Source that has us so blindly attached to dogmas. Ghandi said "Whenever you are confronted with an opponent, conquer him with love." If our true mission in becoming vegan is to save the world from man's destructive behavior, the last thing we need to do is turn our back on man. Like it or not, that man is represented in all of us; he is our mirror, and by not sitting with him at the table, we are showing him the same apathy, aggression, and inhumane behavior vegans once stood against.

On a more tangible note, in April, 2016, one of the most respected and long-standing vegan couples decided to start eating meat: Matthew and Terces Egelhart, owners of popular vegan eateries Gracias Madre and Café Gratitude in California. The public discovery of such a dramatic change in their lifestyle was met with death threats and violence from vegans. They were condemned by popular vegan journals, and longtime clients of their restaurants called them "hypocrites" and "fakers". Matthew and Terces argue that their lifelong purpose is to fix the food system by eradicating violence from the entire system. While living on the farm that produces crops for their restaurants, they observed how every animal has a role in the ecosystem. It was then they realized their intent was to do nothing but let Nature lead the way. As part of this new mission, they started raising livestock, and they intend to manage their farm with the proper use of regenerative agriculture practices in tune with the natural cycles of life*.

The big pink elephant that we fail to see when becoming vegan is the immense responsibility that rests in our shoulders. Just because a product claims to be vegan doesn't mean that it's healthy or that it supports the same ethical beliefs that one stands for. A vegan diet could consist of fake chicken made with soy and wheat, rice contaminated with arsenic, potato chips, Oreos are made with GMO ingredients, and so on. Our responsibility is nothing less than to return to the pace of Nature, cultivate respect towards all living species and Nature's cycles, and take our health back into our own hands. Monocrop agriculture has created a great deal of damage to our forest and jungles; more often than not, these crops occupy the space of hundreds of years old natural flora and fauna, which used to be the habitat of living ecosystems. These crops are being stripped of their soil nutrients because the same crop is grown over and over again without proper crop rotation and cultivation of beneficial bacteria and a natural landscape for native insects and animals. Matthew and Terces Engelhart speak of "regenerative agriculture" where animals coexist with the land:

"Perhaps I've failed to explain adequately why I would pursue the path of eating flesh after 40 years of vegetarianism. The answer is non-violence, but non-violence to the whole system, all species. Agriculture is the most violent destructive force on the planet. (...) Earth Balance margarine is made from Canadian canola. Organic or not, this product required a plow to destroy Canadian prairie, an act of violence against burrowing owls, ferrets, prairie dogs, and dozens of insect and bird species. If that prairie had been maintained in grassland with well managed cows or buffalo those species would not be killed or displaced."

– Terces Engelhart

Maybe the woman on the stage was right, we cannot call vegans plant-based, but we can call all of us plant-based. We come from plants [actually we come from mushrooms], yet we come from the soil and bacteria, and we all return

* http://www.lamag.com/digestblog/gracias-madre-cafe-gratitude-owners-just-pissed-off-entire-vegan-world/

to it. The term plant-based is not meant to segregate people, point fingers, or claim to be the best. Our world is varied enough and the circumstances in which we live are so drastically diverse that due to our different ethnic, cultural, and environmental backgrounds we cannot all eat, live, and think the same way.

If everyone shifted to being plant-based, we would be leaving behind a heavy ecological footprint stigma of petroleum and of disharmony with the environment. It's like asking a lion not to eat a zebra in the jungle. Just as the animal kingdom is varied in its species, we too have differences that limit and dictate our food choices. We need more plant-based choice making, and more plant-based eaters, yes! Yet, we can't demand that up in the Arctic, the natives of that area have the same diet as down in Costa Rica, where abundance of fruit trees and sweet juicy mangoes reigns. Carb-rich sweet fruits have their purpose in the summertime, which is why the trees give fruit during this season and can withstand hot and humid temperatures. Water-rich fruit's purpose is to cool your body down and to help your circadian rhythm adapt by providing high-carb edible pulps, which charge your energy reserves so you can last through the longest daylight days of the year. If someone in the North Pole decided to conduct a fruitarian or raw foods diet, they would literally freeze to death. Rather than cracking the whip on the "ultimate truth" on what diet we should all have, we first must recognize our diversity and understand each socio-individual and bio-individual's needs.

We need one flag we all can wave which will stand for acceptance and respect of all our differences including all living kingdoms. When that time comes, there will be no need to worry about factory farming, because we will know that torturing another living being cannot be justified. Supply and demand will be stable, and you'll change with the environment to adapt to your circumstances, instead of demanding a piece of steak every single night. If a life is given to feed yours, then a moment of appreciation should be one's practice, as a way to show respect to the life that is now a part of you. Bugs won't bother us so much, because we will understand their role in the ecosystem. My daughter calls them "her friends"; she always asks, "where are they going?" or, "where is their home?" When we are all at one with Nature, we will rebuild our future with the Earth, because we can't do it alone. When that time arrives, we will be waving the flag of nourishment, of courage, of generosity, and of respect, because when our intention is in harmony with the fundamental basis of Nature, love will abolish fear, separation, and judgment from the entire universe.

My mission is not to be a vegan, but to inspire others to live in harmony with Nature. It was once my role to be a fundamentalist in order to cross the dark border that had kept me from the truth about health. Once that elementary phase was done, I continued spiraling up through different nourishing phases to align my values or to challenge them and grow. What we all need to do is to see the teachings of different schools of thought from a distance and comprehend the underlying principle of their message.

Honey

Honey has been a favorite food of mine for as long as I can remember. When I visited my grandparents, I would spoon up some of the honey my grandma had bought in "the forests of Quindio or Antioquia". It had a different taste from the honey we used to buy in bear-shaped squeeze bottles. Of course when I first became vegan, the question was; to eat honey or not to eat honey? I was told it was a disgusting act, because honey is "bee's vomit", yet, I never found it gross, but rather interesting. I wondered what the purpose of honey was and how it could benefit our lives. Seen through a different set of eyes, honey is a miracle. Actually, it's not vomit either, it is simply carried by a bee in a gland in its throat and then transferred to another's bee's mouth. This process assures the addition of enzymes to the honey which is collected during this process. Down in Peru, "chicha," their traditional fermented drink, undergoes a similar process. The corn is first chewed by the people in charge of making the drink, then it spit onto the table, then it's left out to ferment. Since the corn has been in contact with the enzymes in the saliva, it guarantees a highly enzymatic fermented drink. This is the traditional way of making *chicha* in the indigenous tribes of the area.

The honey that we most often find in the grocery aisles and in bear-shaped plastic bottles is honey that has been pasteurized, which means heated and stripped of all its medicinal benefits. Honey's characteristics can also be altered when the bees are factory-farmed or are fed high fructose corn syrup. For honey to deliver its healing properties, it has to remain raw and taken from natural pollinators, bees who spend their entire lives foraging in the fields and bringing back nectar from flowers to the hive.

Honey comes with a sizeable quantity of amino acids, which are the protein building blocks we need to survive. It contains B vitamins as well as about 5000 different enzymes, beneficial bacteria, essential nutrients, and antioxidants. Combined with pollen, which is a complete protein and *superfood* [which can be consumed by humans as well as bees], it's what keeps a bee healthy, energetic, and strong throughout its life. Although what I find most interesting is how honey can be used as an antibacterial, internally and externally. Biochemist Peter Charles Molan of New Zealand has found in his research that honey reacts with the body's fluids to make hydrogen peroxide, creating an inhospitable environment for bacteria[*]. If you ever wondered why we cannot feed honey to infants under 1 year of age, it's not because they might choke with the viscose substance as one might think, it's due to the antibacterial properties of honey, which are so powerful that it can harm the young and delicately forming microbiome in the babies' bodies.

Bees need our help. Just last year in 2015, 42% of the bee population in the U.S died[**]. That's outrageous! The common causes are pesticide use, global warming, loss of habitat, and disease. A week or so ago, when the Zika mosquito infestation in Miami occurred, pesticides were sprayed throughout our city and surrounding fields. Even in Zika free zones like South Carolina, small airplanes rained Naled onto the farms without properly warning the farmers and animal keepers. 2.5 million Bees died instantly just in that area. Without bees there is no pollination – bees pollinate 100 different human food crops, which provide around 90 percent of the world's nutrition.[***]Without bees there would be no flowers or trees; without trees there would be no home for small animals and without them, there's no planetary ecosystem. Bees have been on the planet for 27 million years, performing the job of pollination and honey-making for their entire existence. It is said that their society is structured to perfection. And yet, bees' lives are now threatened as we start messing up the perfect Nature of things. To this day there are seven species of bees in danger of extinction.

When voting with our dollars, these are the kinds of factors we have to consider to truly benefit the greater cause. It's not a personal ethical issue but a global one. Not buying raw honey from local beekeepers is failing to support individuals who have dedicated their lives to properly setting up home for bees. Although it takes 300 bees three weeks to make an ounce of honey, they create enough extra for moderate human consumption. Raw honey is the product exchange in which abundance comes to the farmers for having promoted life from the bottom of the chain of life up. We need to support local, sustainable agriculture; we need the bees as much as they need our protection from our careless destruction.

During recent lectures I was giving on Our Relationship with Food, when it's time for questions, often *veganism* is what draws a lot of interest. I make vegan people uncomfortable when I speak of raw dairy or honey. I often see confusion in their faces. I know what they are feeling. I've been there. I had my measures of balance while I was transitioning to eating vegan. However what I carelessly became attached to for some time, was not so much maintaining a zero animal byproducts policy, but an obsession with eating healthy. It's called "orthorexia", and it's an eating issue. Orthorexia is when we become obsessed with eating a certain way, but that's just a surface symptom. Often food disorders come up as a reminder of something deeper that's happening in our emotional bodies. We often take our relationship with food as a religious doctrine in order to instill structure or a sense of guidance in our lives. We are looking for answers, or expecting something else to captain our boat, so that we can let go of the steering wheel and live on autopilot. At other times, our aim for perfection may come from a self-

*   https://draxe.com/the-many-health-benefits-of-raw-honey/
**   https://www.nrdc.org/stories/buzz-about-colony-collapse-disorder?gclid=CjoKEQjwjem-BRC_isGJIJ-oh-
MBEiQAbCimWLfbnw_FIJLAulm34Yq4amG692U2ugdkBtCnFj_Wy-kaAlk38P8HAQ
***   http://www.onegreenplanet.org/news/swarm-of-bees-follows-queen-trapped-in-car/

limiting belief of not being enough, or of wanting to control something when we lack control of everything else around us. For me, it was a combination of all of the above. I was going through a rough emotional rollercoaster with my daughter's father. Our relationship was on the edge; I didn't want to do the necessary thing when it came time to end it, thus not taking responsibility for my life. I thought very poorly of myself, and therefore felt inadequate, and everything around me seemed to bring chaos, which gave me the urge to look for any way I could control things! Marc David, founder of the Psychology of Eating Institute, explains this phenomenon of reaching for food when chaos overruns our lives as a search for nourishment and a "safe" place to hide. Our first understanding of nourishment and of being safe goes back to our earliest days, when we received our first taste of milk from our moms. Milk, which was the food that nourished us, meant love, meant being taken care of, meant being safe in our mother's arms. Every food disorder we deal with, from anorexia and bulimia to binge eating and chronic dieting, has a symbolic meaning pointing to an empty or unfulfilled emotion inside us.

In life we go through different phases. Back in the 1960's, psychologist of the time concluded that we initiate a new chapter in our lives every seven years, so it is in our social and psychological makeup to live our lives in segments. Whatever growth path you are on, you will find that to progress from A to B, there's a stage that teaches us how to get to B. For instance, there are five stages of grief: denial, anger, bargaining, depression, and acceptance. By the same token, we have ten phases of Nourishment related to how we eat. In no particular order, they are: cleansing, building, sustaining, the emotional phase, celebration, learning, the fundamental phase, healing, surrender, the trickster phase, and the death phase.

We are not supposed to become stagnant or attached to any of these phases; they are part of our learning curve as we move through life and explore our own wisdom – how to get from A to B. These phases are also a reflection of where we stand on our path. Becoming obsessed about or blinded by something, whether it is a phase or another person, is closing your door to what tomorrow has prepared for you.

Kraut

If I were to ask you what the biggest threat to humanity is, how many guesses would it take for you to say antibiotic-resistant bacteria? Even more than nuclear bombs, terrorism, climate change, or war, pathogens could destroy the entire human race and every living organism in a short period of time. Vani Hari, better known as the Food Babe, shared this fact during one of her lectures. Her talk was part of a conference called Longevity led by David Wolfe. To my surprise, during the conference bacteria was the most urgent topic addressed by every single speaker no matter their expertise, from how to support good bacteria to warnings against the dangerous kind. This included the likes of Dr. Mercola, Nadine Artemis, and David Asprey from the Bulletproof diet. All of them, as well as many current leaders in the medical field, unanimously argue that the inclusion of probiotics is the number one intervention we can implement to improve our health.

Bacteria play an essential role in our survival. They outnumber us by far. Out of every 10 cells in your body, 9 of them belong to bacteria. So it is fair to say that we are 90% bacteria and 10% human. You can find about 300 million bacteria in a kiss, and other 300 trillion bacteria residing in your body. However, we need to make an important distinction when speaking about bacteria, and we need to understand how the bacterial world operates, to prevent mistaken assumptions. A bacterium is a microscopic single-cell organism that spends its life growing and dividing itself at an exponential rate. Since bacteria live in our bodies, they have a synergetic and vital relationship with us. The bacteria found in our intestines, which are called the microbiome or intestinal flora, are what account for our proper digestion. Bacteria are in fact the organisms that digest our food, specifically fiber; they absorb and retain nutrients for us and keep pathogens at bay. Also, bacteria provide essential vitamins such as B12 as well as enzymes in substances they excrete. On the surface of our bodies, bacteria create an invisible shield to protect us from harmful outside bacteria.

If you wonder why vegans usually are deficient in vitamin B12, it is due to the lack of probiotics in their diet. People who eat meat or eggs get their B12 from those foods. In a cow's stomach there are bacteria that helps the cow digest food and that release essential vitamins like B12. Since this process is symbiotic, we absorb these vitamins from other living animals, and we can't absorb them from vegetables, although we can from unwashed organic produce or contact with dirt, and by eating fermented foods or taking a probiotic supplement. B vitamins are essential for our proper functioning; they provide us with energy and also help us absorb iron.

The 21st century is dealing with the consequences of one of the major 20th century creations: Antibiotics. This scientific advance to eliminate deadly infections by creating an antibiotic that will target bacteria was a sensation at the time. Many lives were saved due to the introduction of this stellar medical discovery. However, as time went on, bacteria continued their rapid genetic evolution by recreating itself with new resistance to the antibiotic that killed the previous generation.

The field of scientific research on bacteria is quite new, even though bacteria existed before any other living being on the planet. They have been around for billions of years, and yet we have not been able to figure them entirely. We have a dozen million bacteria in our gut, and yet we can only acknowledge a few. However, what we eventually discovered was that by repeated use of antibacterial medications, we not only killed the bad bacteria, but the good bacteria as well. With no beneficial bacteria protecting us, we are vulnerable to new viral threats, to other pathogens, and to every new contagious disease. There are brief TED talks on the subjects of bacterial reproduction and antibiotic-resistant bacteria by biochemists Bonnie Bassler and Karl Klose, who explain this information in detail. We also have pesticide-, fungicide-, and insecticide-resistant bacteria, and bacteria resistant even to toxic man-manipulated chemicals. If we can't kill pathogenic bacteria, we are at *exponential* risk.

The use of pesticides and GMO products present a farther threat to our wellbeing. It's not only the cancers, autism cases, digestive issues, and endocrine and neurological breakdowns we've seen due to eating genetically modified foods, it's what we haven't seen yet. GMO encoding is being absorbed by bacteria, and in the process of division and cellular growth, they become new GMO bacterial organisms and penetrate and change our genetic code too. If we are spray pesticides on our soil, harmful chemical-resistant bacteria are being carried from seed to our table. If you eat meat and do not take care where it is coming from, even more antibacterial-resistant substances are passing from cow to steak to your plate. 80% of all antibacterial pharmaceuticals used are being given to factory farm animals. These animals become sicker and sicker after being removed from their natural environments, more new viruses and infections are spreading, and it is all landing in your gut.

However, new studies are showing how bacteria are receptive not only to harm but also to good. For instance, bacteria can be turned into beneficial by simply playing classical music around them, or sticking an "I love you" label on the jar. Bacteria respond not only to our actions but also our thoughts! Candida yeast, for example, is a very common problem in women. One of the root reasons these organism turns against us is stress. Remember, stress is the body's response to any threat, whether *imaginary* or real.

Perhaps you've heard about the work of Japanese doctor Masaru Emoto. His research focused on water molecules and how they respond to the environment around them. Just as bacteria do, water changes its form according to our current expression. If 70% of our body is water and 90%

(or 99%, if our genetic code is taken into consideration) is bacteria, we are receptive to every single thing that surrounds us, even glimpsed thoughts as well as what we hear and see feeds or nourishes us on a certain level: a song on the radio, a horror movie or a comedy, a good deep conversation or a screaming fight all have an effect. Imagine the power of meditation!

Instead of just looking the other way, we need to keep digging into these discoveries. There is a natural rhythm of things. The world contracts and expands, just as we inhale and exhale. It's a constant progression of time. Our exhale moment came when we found the cure to some things, but everything has a life span, and that includes our antibiotics, our vaccines, our values, our diets, even how we look at the world. We once thought the world was flat, didn't we? We have to keep shifting. We must inhale again, and continue to reinvent ourselves. That's what bacteria have been doing for billions of years, maybe there's a lesson to be learned from them... We must keep adapting to change.

Nutritionally speaking, we have an immediate answer that can help us help *ourselves*. In most ancient cultures fermentation was used in some way or other. Korea has kimchi, Peru has *chicha*, Egypt discovered sourdough, the French have cheese. Wine and beer are products of fermented fruits, grains, or sugar, and even chocolate is a fermented manjar. Fermented foods in ancient times were considered a divine miracle; how else could people then explain that a food could become better after its death by means invisible to the human eye? It's almost poetic to talk about fermenting foods. Fermenting foods are decomposing matter being eaten by minuscule single-cell organisms called bacteria or yeast. Just as bacteria excrete nutrients and enzymes in our digestive systems, the same is happening to a piece of cabbage, or to the combination of wheat, water, and salt when making traditional sourdough. When enjoying these sour foods, we are inadvertently helping our intestinal flora to flourish. It's popular now to take probiotic supplements of strains such as acidophilus, saccharomyces, bifidus, or lactobacillus in the form of pills. The probiotic colony in each pill is only 5-10 million organisms. However, when consuming fermented foods like Kombucha (fermented tea), yogurt, or sauerkraut, each bite or sip of these foods can provide us with 300 million different beneficial colonies. Beneficial bacteria are also susceptible to heat, so fermented foods to remain medicinal must be eaten raw.

If your doctor prescribes you an antibiotic, the proper way to take it is to follow it with a probiotic. Ask your doctor what the active time frame of the antibiotic is, then when its active cycle is done, take your probiotic. That way once you purge any dangerous bacteria from your system, you can resupply your intestines with friendly bacteria.

Once again, I'm convinced our health can be improved right from our own kitchen. It's in our hands to create our own medicine by simply taking in a piece of Nature. Some things must keep evolving, including all human creations. Yet Nature was perfected before us, and so was the universe. We must keep tuning onto and aligning ourselves with their rhythm.

Seasons

Rhythm is action. It's a step above balance, and far beyond moderation. I've learned to not even include "moderation" in my lexicon. If I do, it's a sign telling me to take back control of the situation. Most times when we leave it up to "moderation", that is saying let someone else decide for you. It is feeling too comfortable to do anything. It is simply letting go of the rope and living a completely monotonous and unchallenging life.

Rhythm is attractive. It is acknowledging the presence of two parallel but opposite forces; it's a dance. It is the yin and yang.

Nature has its own rhythm, turning from spring to winter. The world rotates365 times a year, constantly revolving around the sun. We are born and we die. Reishi, the queen of mushrooms and medicinal herbs, is born at the beginning stages of a birch forest. Chaga, the king of mushrooms and medicinal herbs, grows at the final decaying phase of the birch trees. Everything seems to be in synchronicity, the hibernation of a bear during winter, or the birds waking with the sunrise. Even the lioness is in rhythm when hunting, performing her dance only once a week. Our circadian rhythm proves that we too are married to this silent heartbeat of the earth; however, when it comes to instinctively aligning with the nature of things, we are deaf to this universal pulse.

We already know fruits are abundant in summer to cool down our bodies and to provide us with energy from their high carbohydrate content. Coconuts populate our beaches in hot climates to recharge us and provide us with natural electrolytes. At the same time, during fall, winter, and spring, we can tune ourselves to the music of Nature to find the proper foods to bring to our table.

As each season begins it sets the tone for what our diet should be. During fall and winter, nuts and grains that dictate a high fat, high protein diet keeps us warm and full for longer periods of time; in spring, there's an abundance of greens and sprouts, hence low fat, highly bitter foods and a low humidity diet provide us with a time for cleansing; and during summer, fruits supply us with a high carb diet for more energy during the longer sunny days. John Douillard, expert on Ayurveda and Western Medicine, explains in his 3-Season Diet book how each one of these seasonal eating habits are oddly the same trendy diets other medical leaders are trying to encourage upon us; they do so, however, with the blinding concept of doing one "seasonal diet" for the rest of our lives. The disharmony caused by eating as one should in winter all year long triggers our biology to naturally crave carbs, sugars, or whatever food group we are not getting enough of. Furthermore, it will create a state where starvation is signaled by the way of your diet, which suggests the stress of a possible food shortage or famine to your body. By now, you know that this kind of anxiety causes stress in your body, which leads to the your sympathetic nervous system retaining fat, and shutting down digestion in order to prevent starvation and improper use of energy reserves.

Diets don't work, because they are phases that try to change your life no matter the health circumstances, environmental conditions, or emotional burdens. Common fad diets are oblivious to the rhythm of things; they constantly play a tune that soon becomes an annoying ear-worm, which eventually drives you crazy, i.e., cravings, imbalance, improper digestion, gaining weight back, and lack of energy.

We've created a new eating craze. Our society now is populated by chronic-dieting victims, who walk around feeling guilty or inadequate for some 20 or even 40 years of their lives. We often compare ourselves to the guy next door, or to the woman on that magazine cover. We get stuck on one answer. We want nothing but to fix our problems the same way that "everyone" else does – or that we think they do. I don't believe we are broken, but we have been sidetracked. The need to "fix" things, to fit in, and to stay the same is what harms us the most. There's no one answer for everyone, because we are diverse individuals, our social interactions are varied, our belief systems are different, our bodies are different, and our energy is recharged by different inspirational sources. In a way, we all have our own spring to winter phases; we all have our own innate rhythm. After looking for the answers outside of ourselves, we need to look within. There's a time to accept gaining weight andslowing down, a time for reflection being a bit more introverted, and even a time to fall down and stay on the bottom for a bit. Chronic dieters are usually people who refuse to change, or better said, are afraid of change. They need to have predictable lunches and dinners and count calories. Their stability is based on numbers and sizes. Their lives are methodical and fueled by the fear of uncertainty.

The only universal rule that applies to all of us is change. Change may mean we are getting older, or our hips are getting bigger, or our babies are now talking, or our grandparents are slowing down. Change may mean I'm wiser than last year, or quieter, or living in a different house. Change means expansion, it is growth. The rhythm of things, the rhythm of Nature and of our heartbeat invites us to let go and trust the uncertainty and unpredictability life has to offer us.

Seasonal Vegetables

Best are highlighted in color
Adapted from John Douillard's *The 3-Season Diet*, pg. 109

Spring

Tangy Apples	Collard Greens
Blueberries	Corn
Dried Fruits	Dandelions
Grapefruit	Endive
Lemons	Fennel
Limes	Garlic
Papayas	Ginger
Pears	Green Beans
Pomegranates	Hot Peppers
Raspberries	Jicama
Strawberries	Kale
Alfalfa Sprouts	Leeks
Artichokes	Lettuce
Asparagus	Mushrooms
Bean Sprouts	Mustard Greens
Beets	Onions
Bell Peppers	Parsley
Broccoli	Peas
Brussels Sprouts	Snow Peas
Cabbage	Baked Potatoes
Carrots	Seaweed
Cauliflower	Spinach
Celery	Swiss Chard
Chicory	Radishes
Dried Chili Peppers	Turnips
Cilantro	Watercress

Summer

Apples
Apricots
Bananas
Blueberries
Cantaloupes
Cherries
Coconuts
Cranberries
Dates
Dried Fruits
Figs
Grapes
Guavas
Mangoes
Melons
Nectarines
Sweet Oranges
Papayas
Tree-Ripened Peaches
Pears
Persimmons
Pineapples
Plums
Pomegranates
Raspberries
Strawberries
Sweet Tangerines
Alfalfa Sprouts
Artichokes
Asparagus
Avocados
Bean Sprouts
Bell Peppers
Broccoli

Cabbage
Cauliflower
Celery
Chicory
Cilantro
Collard Greens
Corn
Cucumbers
Dandelions
Eggplant
Endive
Fennel
Green Beans
Jicama
Kale
Lettuce
Mushrooms
Mustard Greens
Okra
Cooked Onions
Parsley
Peas
Potatoes
Pumpkins
Seaweed
Spinach (in moderation)
Acorn Squash
Winter Squash
Sweet Potatoes
Swiss Chard
Tomatoes (in moderation)
Watercress
Zucchini

Winter

Cooked apples	Tangerines
Apricots	Avocados
Bananas	Beets
Blueberries	Brussels sprouts
Cantaloupe	Carrots
Cherries	Chili Peppers
Coconut (ripe)	Corn
Cranberries	Eggplant
Dates	Fennel
Figs	Garlic
Grapefruit	Ginger
Grapes	Hot Peppers
Guava	Cooked Kale
Lemons	Leeks
Limes	Okra
Mangoes	Onions
Nectarines	Parsley
Oranges	Mashed Potatoes
Papayas	Pumpkin
Peaches	Cooked Seaweed
Ripe Pears	Acorn Squash
Persimmons	Winter Squash
Pineapples	Sweet Potatoes
Plums	Tomatoes
Strawberries	Turnips

Nourishing Path

- What do you admire about a plant-based diet?
- What nourishing path do are you on right now?
- What do you think you can do to improve your work/home environment, and thus reduce stress?

Nourishing Tips

- Practice a random act of self-love every day
- Take at least 20 minutes to complete your meals, especially if you are stressed
- Take 3 to 5 deep breaths before eating
- Give thanks for your food, or create your own prayer before a meal
- Get 7-8 hours of sleep
- Get out in the sun at least 10 minutes a day
- Try switching from a mainstream detergent or soap brand to an eco-friendly one
- Support a local farmer by buying local sustainably-harvested raw honey
- Make your own sauerkraut

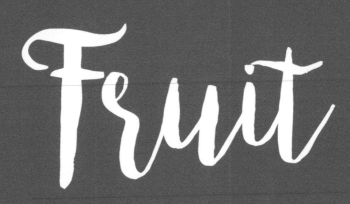

"If you really want to make a friend, go to someone's house and eat with him... The people who give you their food, give you their heart."

— Cesar Chavez

Chopsticks

Today's Special is an independent film about a young French-trained chef. The plot revolves around how this young chef sees his culture as a limitation to practicing his art. He is from India, and his father owns an Indian restaurant in New York. He wants to serve French food, not *chicken masala.* Eventually, his father gets sick, and the young chef is forced to manage the restaurant in his absence. He solves his dilemma by merging the two cultures he loves, the one that is in his blood, and the one that has grown in his heart. The movie talks about culture, art, and tradition, and it has one line that I'll never forget: "Eating with a fork and knife is like making love through an interpreter." In India's Hindu culture, food is commonly eaten with the hands.

In Morocco, food is served in beautiful clay pots called *tajines.* It's traditional to sit around the table and have someone walk around to wash your hands before and after dinner. Their philosophy is based on gathering around one round tray, where there's no head of the table and no foot. A common saying goes: "Eat with one finger and you are selfish, if you eat with two fingers you are more caring, but if you eat with three fingers you are generous." The number of fingers you use represents how delicious you think the food is and how grateful you are for it. The round table, sharing the same plate, and eating with the hands culturally symbolizes equality at the table, love of sharing, and bringing family, friends, and guests together. Eating is about community.

In certain countries in Africa they also eat with their hands. The universal method of doing so is to keep the right hand for eating and the left hand for anything not associated with food. You usually take food from each sharing tray on the side closest to you. This protocol allows everyone to eat with their hands in a peaceful systematic way.

In China, it was Confucius who inspired the use of chopsticks at the table rather than a knife or fork: "The honorable and upright man keeps well away from both the slaughterhouse and the kitchen. And he allows no knives on his table." Silverware at the table symbolized violence. This tradition then extended to other Asian nations.

How can these traditions translate to our current times? The overall message is simply to slow down.

I recently had the pleasure of coming across the work of Sarah Linda Ferror. She's a product designer from Amsterdam who has created a collection of seven utensils. Each eating tool is shaped into a rustic, organic rustic figure. Picture an oyster's shell, yet every tool has sensuous concave and delicate curves like a leaf. Her work brings us closer to our food by taking us into a new way of experiencing eating, where eating itself is its own form of art. She states:

"Not being cutlery nor plates, these tools evoke in us a more intuitive way of eating, giving new value to our food. They transform the act of eating into a moment of full attention, gratefulness, and pleasure."

The top advice I can give to anyone who has digestive issues of any kind is simply to slow down. Our mechanistic ways of eating and detachment from our food is causing disassociation from what food should be, and from our own lives.

Food, which our society depends on for financial, economic, and social support, is actually only here to nurture us.

Kitchen

So eating and cooking are a cultural thing. That means there is information in your next bite. If there was no culture, how could we claim to be a society? By losing our cooking skills, we are losing much more than a warm plate on the table. We are losing history, wisdom, tradition, and nourishment. Perhaps this is what differentiates us from the rest of the animal kingdom. It's not our evolved thinking, or amazing communication skills, or technological advances – it can be argued that we aren't the real pioneers as far as "advancements" when there are ancient creatures that have developed the ability to communicate using echolocation, or to produce their own light via bioluminescence. What distinguishes us from the rest of the living world is our ability to tell a story.

We tell stories through art, and some stories are told through food. Humanity has been evolving for about seven million years, according to anthropological findings. Through these ages we have had to adapt to our circumstances. Cooking has evolved since the discovery of fire, however, one thing remains the same; we've always had and will continue to have a need to eat.

In Michael Pollan's documentary series "Cooked" on Netflix, he points out the interesting position of the cook in our culture; on one side we have those who we feed, and on the other we have the source of those foods: Nature. The cook is almost a passage for information from Nature to humanity.

The cook is a storyteller, an interpreter, an entertainer, a mother, and a teacher. But this bridge is being threatened by industrialization. If we eradicate cooks from our culture, as we have already been seeing, our human race will descend into chaos. There will be no orchestra conductor, no rhythm, no balance of supply and demand, no connection with the earth, and no understanding of us being part of this living world if that happens.

As soon as industrialization came in and presented its solution to the problem of feeding the masses, we started getting sick. Our foods contained more processed sugar than fat, fats were hydrogenated and impossible to digest, and junk food penetrated our houses as black mold that won't go away. Factory farming was introduced to meet consumer demand for one dollar cheeseburgers, and now our kids are becoming obese, even newborns.

We have lost control of our appetites, of our portions, of the times when we eat, of eating seasonally and intuitively, and of our health. Sadly, this story is reflected collectively in current levels of cooking skills.

A society that doesn't eat will perish. A culture that has no culinary focus is lost. A world without cooks is like homes without mothers. Cooking is a feminine energy role. Even the toughest, manliest cook has this quality within him. To cook is to nourish.

I'm an advocate for plant-based living. I believe this lifestyle has a way of infiltrating our minds and changing our nutritional beliefs, to the benefit and overall health of our minds, bodies, and souls. Yet beyond the tangible aspects of this way of eating is the underlying principle of coming home to our inner and outer Nature. I accept and celebrate our diversity, and understand that the entire world cannot be herbivorous; however, we can all become more aware, more awake to our surroundings, more understanding, and more compassionate to those who are different from us. I'm not only speaking of species recognition, but of eliminating racism, nationalism, fanaticism, and ego-driven stereotypical structures.

It might be that cooking, like any other art form, is a way of rebellion. It's a need for movement filtered into an energy of creation. What we are rebelling against is that dormant self that has lost touch with what its purpose is. We are all here to emanate respect toward all phases of life, even death. We are here to give thanks for our existence and celebrate it. When we nourish our bodies, we are being responsible for our own wellbeing and everyone else's on the planet.

How can you learn to cook? Simple. Google, my friends. There's a recipe for everything. There's so many ways to crack an egg! Can you cook? Answer these questions, and if you respond, "Yes" to any of them, you can cook.

Have you traveled outside your home, to a different town, city, or country?

Do you live in a household with loved ones?

Do you love food?

That's what it takes to cook. Culture, memories, and love.

Relationship with Food

We are emotional beings. We are in constant motion, which is sparked by our feelings. All we desire, all we do is so that we will feel a certain way. Too often we try to fix ourselves with a straightforward solution. The problem is, such a remedy will give us a "quick fix" burst of instant feelings, but those emotions will then disperse into the ether as fast as they came. If we want a lasting solution, a body that suits us, and an authentic smile, we have to understand our problems are not so quickly solved. Just as we need a *functional practitioner* doctor to treat us when we are not feeling well, and as the doctor will look at the overall behavior of our organs, systems, and symptoms, we have to study ourselves from this same tridimensional perspective.

We are not just physical; we are mind, body, and spirit. We are emotional beings who perceive the world and are fed through our five senses. Hence, our relationship with food is much deeper than what we just see served on the plate.

We eat through what we observe, what we choose to hear, what we feel, what we touch and how we touch; we eat what we taste and through what we say to others and to ourselves. In the end, what's served on the plate is irrelevant, if the intention of eating is reduced to simply eating because you have to. We need to eat for love, for pleasure, for kindness. We have to eat for quality, and raise the bar of what we believe we deserve, and demand it.

The solution to our diet dilemmas, our lifestyles, and our illnesses requires a nourishing energy, an energy that is soft, gentle, and patient. We need to tenderly tend our wounds like a mother and embrace more of our feminine energy, which is present in both men and women. We need to cook!

My intention in explaining my views and what I have gathered on this path of culinary studies, food counseling, and nutrition is to offer an invitation to think about food in a different way. The main lesson plant-based eating has taught me is one of awareness, presence, and community. Choose your next meal with these principles, and you'll be *nourishing* and aligning your inner mind–body–soul trinity with the All.

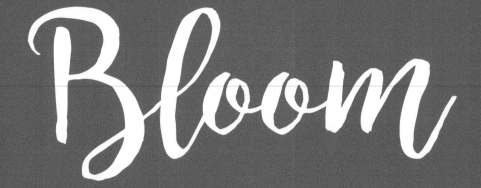

"Abundance: the ability to do what you need to do, when you need to do it."

— Bashar

Nourished

After writing my first chapter, I hit a brick wall. I didn't know how I could write a book about healing your body when mine was back on a road to destruction. I discovered I had Hashimoto's thyroiditis. Hashimoto's is an autoimmune disease where the body attacks itself. In essence, my body created antibodies which were attacking my thyroid. Hashimoto's is a chronic hypothyroid condition. The difference between hypothyroid and Hashimoto's diagnoses is the presence of antibodies, mineral deficiencies, and the production of thyroid cells. The symptoms are still quite similar. Fatigue was the main symptom bringing me down.

However, after being forced to slow down due to my ongoing exhaustion, I stepped back and took a look at my life from a distance. I recognized that I had left out all the values that I consistentlystand for. My work had become my obsession and a shield to numb my feelings away. Instead of cooking, I was eating the leftovers of what I'd prepared for my daughter; I had no schedule for lunch, and I was living in a constant rush.

But I refused to be a "victim" of anything. I started reading books on all aspects of healing and did research to understand the physiological makeup of the thyroid. My first revelation was that a thyroid imbalance is just another symptom. The organ itself is not broken, it's just trying to protect us by borrowing something from another organ or gland, causing and ongoing domino effect of imbalances throughout the body. Like a detective I traced down my symptoms, my emotions, my situations with work, money, and relationships, and I discovered the root cause of my condition. In the field of functional medicine is called Chronic Fatigue, in my words is lack of [self] love, and a mandatory need to slow down. During my journey when I started healing my hyperthyroid back in 2013, I was able to balance my hormones and bring my hyperthyroid symptoms back to normal during my pregnancy. I had done it for my daughter. My need to achieve health was for her sake. She was a beautiful light of inspiration, which I kept hold of to bring me out of the depths of my ruin.

This time around, I had to do it for me. Now I have to thank my thyroid for offering me the challenge of understanding it, of understanding myself, and of once more proving that every single visible symptom is just a signal of inner emotional turmoil. My Hashimoto's thyroiditis forced me to slow down. When we slow down, we start discovering the beauty of every single minuscule thing that stands in front of us, and we simply fall in love with the world. In a way, slowing down is a forced path to a total humbling gratitude.

My Hashimoto's brought me back home to thank my mother [who was vital in my path to healing], and to my love for cooking. It brought me home to appreciate the earth and my new daily morning walks with my dog. It brought me back to slowing down during mealtimes, choosing my foods more wisely, and noticing which foods helped the most. It made me appreciate going back to swimming in the ocean and wanting to sleep in a little bit longer. Hashimoto's reminded me there's something beautiful about breathing, about being in a body, and standing here with my shoulders back and my heart upright. My thyroid simply reminded me of my voice and of my mission: to nourish the world, including myself.

I have my condition to thank for being the inspiration to write this book. After breathing, writing, and practicing my own advice, I was able to lower the level of my autoimmune condition, yet I'm still on my healing path.

Our best teachers are usually disguised as what we think are our worst enemies. What or who do you have to thank today?

#Nourishedpath

My favorite lecturer and author is Marianne Williamson; I often reach into her books for guidance. In her book *A Return to Love*, she invites us all to make a shift of perspective. In the realm of society, partnership, and friendship, instead of saying "You and me against the world", she suggests that we don't get into [partnership] to escape the world, we get married to heal the world together.

I was once invited to be a guest on a podcast to discuss my path to eating vegan. The first thing we discussed was the feeling of belonging I felt when I discovered that way of thinking. But it was never absent, it was always here, even before I experienced it. That sense of cameraderie, togetherness, and sharing is embedded in all of us. We are all connected before conception; we are an energy that inspires progress and creation. It's in the moment when we want to isolate ourselves that this energy can become destructive.

If you want to practice a plant-based lifestyle and you feel excluded from your family or friends, change your perspective. You are simply in a different growth phase, which is part of your path to teach you, to heal you, or to simply challenge you.

You are never alone. We are healing the world together.

I want to invite you, the reader, to interact with me and with others on the path of nourishing their lives by connecting via social media through the *hashtag* #nourishedpath. We can exchange recipes, thoughts, frustrations, and triumphs and have an ongoing platform for our ever-evolving path.

Thank YOU for being here.

Nourished Tips

Below is a list of practical actions we can do on a daily, weekly, or monthly basis to enrich our lives on a nourished way. Of course, the more you practice, the quicker the change of mindset, for a more relaxed, happy and nurtured life.

Meditate at least 10 minutes a day. You can find guided meditations on YouTube and then simply play them on your phone while you are in a relaxed position focusing on your breath. Pedram Shojai has audio breathing meditations on his website, Well.org. Marianne Williamson and Deepak Chopra also offer free videos on YouTube. If you simply want to listen to relaxing music, search on apps like Spotify or Pandora for meditation tracks.

Take a walk in the morning, evening, or at night. If you take your walk after the sunlit hours, make sure to spend at least 10 minutes in the sun, either after lunch or have breakfast on your porch. If walking is not an option for you, you can asit under the sky and apply breathing techniques while relaxing on a reclining chair.

Take 3-5 deep breaths before you eat. This helps you by grounding you before eating and sets the tone for your body to welcome the food. By pumping air deep into your abdomen, you are activating better digestion and proper assimilation.

Give thanks for your food, either mentally or aloud. You can say a prayer, a simple "thank you" or *bon appetit.* Thank the cook, thank the earth, or thank the food and the moment. You can also thank any prescription medicine or herb to receive its healing properties.

Slow down when you eat. Eat with chopsticks, or if the setting allows it, eat with your hands!

Have your biggest portion of food at lunchtime between noon and 2:30pm. Eat before sunset.

Lower or turn off as many artificial lights as possible after sunset. Get a red bulb for a small lamp in your room. Or a Himalayan salt lamp! Light candles perfumed with relaxing essential oils like lavender around your house, and try to limit the use of electronics 2-3 hours before bed.

Replace mainstream brands of body soaps with alternative, eco-friendly, mineral based products.

Visit a farmers market. Buy organic and local if possible.
Include more fermented foods in your diet.
If not plant-based, go Meatless on Mondays.
Cook for your loved ones – that includes you!
Treat yourself.
Enjoy your food! Play!
Always ask *why?*

Conclusion

"...just because you were not writing externally does not mean you were not writing internally."

- Nayyirah Waheed

I wrote this book about *our* nature. Our natural state, which is always changing.

This book is about change, about the different phases that we go through towards evolution or destruction. It's about beauty, but not the one we see but the one we can feel.

There's beauty in birth, in growth, and in death. Beauty surrounds us wherever Nature is present it's the message that is here to speak to us. Nothing lasts, nothing stays the same, we can't bottle a blooming sunflower, but in completing the stages of our growth, we will always blossom stronger, wiser, and kinder. That's the beauty of living.

We also go through phases with our diet. My message is not to be fanatical about any doctrine, but to tune into the rhythm of life, of the moment, and of our emotions, and morph with it.

Change.

The only constant.

Plant-Based

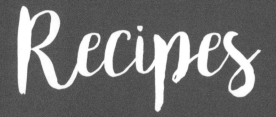
Recipes

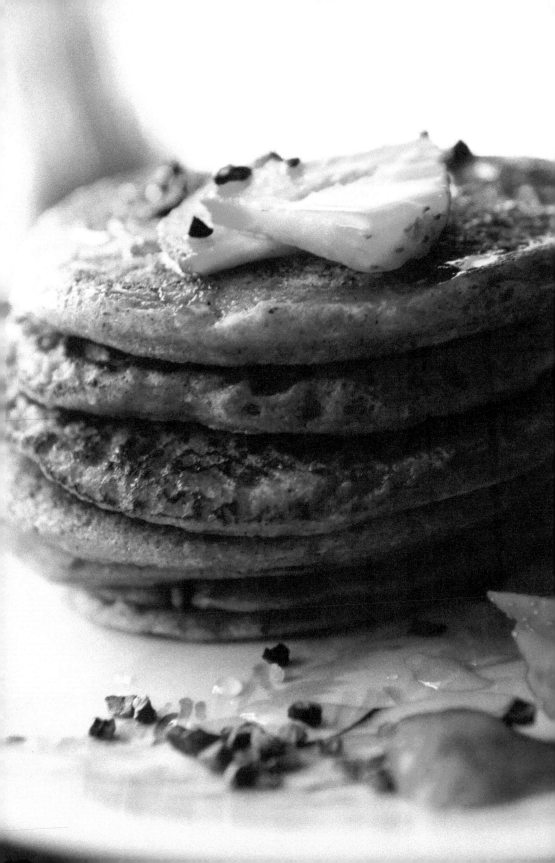

Pancakes

Ingredients

Makes 7
Portion: one quarter cup

- ¼ Cup Golden Flax Meal
- ½ Cup Brown Rice Flour
- ¼ Cup + 2 Tbsp of Oat Flour
- 2 Tbsp Coconut Oil, melted
- 2 Tbsp Natural Maple Syrup
- ¼ Tsp Mineral Salt
- ½ Tsp Baking Soda
- 1 Cup Rice Milk or Nut Milk
- ½ Tsp Vanilla Powder or 1 Tsp of Vanilla Extract

Directions

- Set aside a skillet for your pancakes; warm it over low heat while you prepare the batter.

- In a medium size bowl, whisk all dry ingredients together. It's important to whisk it before adding liquid ingredients to avoid clumps. Then add liquid ingredients.

- If your coconut oil is solid, measure what you need and pour it over a glass cup, then melt in your toaster oven for 2–3 minutes. You can also run warm water over the whole jar of coconut oil, or simply measure what you need and melt in a skillet. Once melted, add to the dry ingredients bowl.

- Add maple syrup, milk, and vanilla.
- Continue whisking vigorously. The batter will thicken as you let it sit. That's okay. You can always add a bit more milk or water.

- Turn the stove up to medium high. It's important for the stove to be really hot for the pancakes to come out right, which is why I always warm up the pan while I prepare my batter.

- You can use a ¼ cup measure to pour the batter over the pan. Once the batter looks set, flip the pancake. It takes about 2–3 minutes per side.

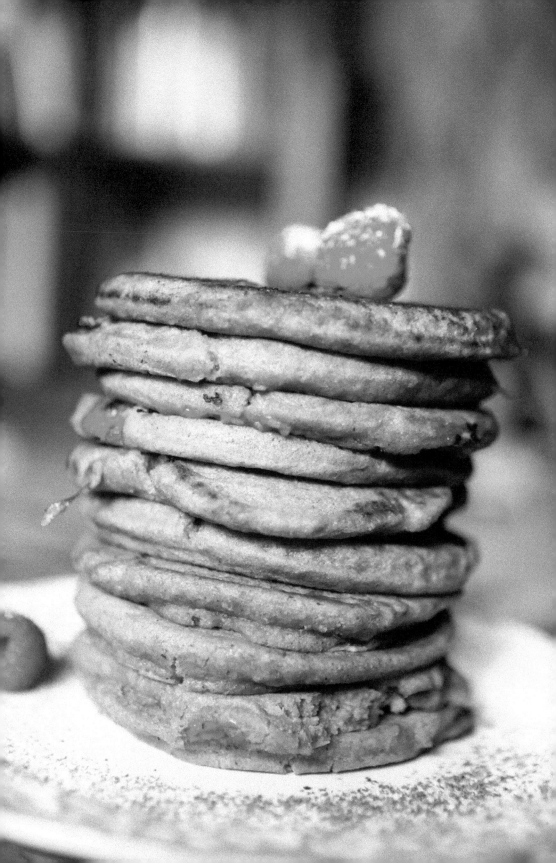

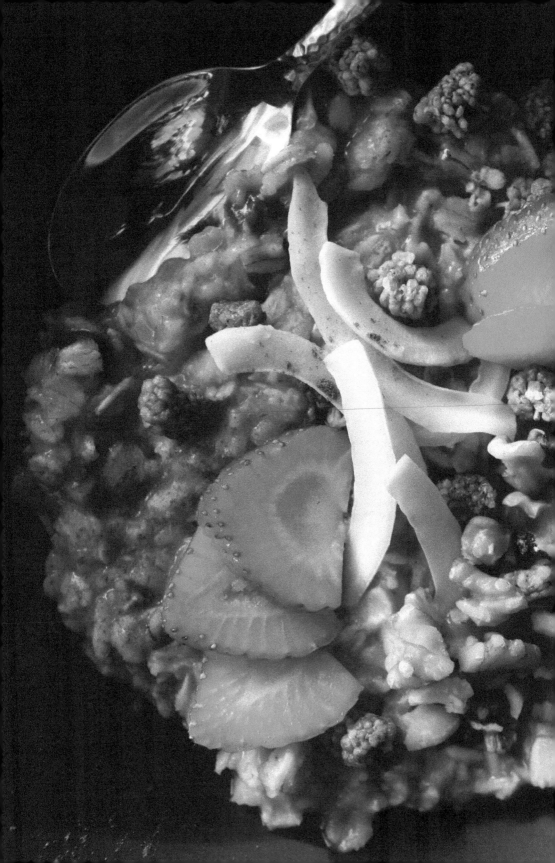

Oatmeal

Ingredients

Makes 2
Portion: one cup

- 1 Cup Rice Milk
- 1/8 tsp Ground Cinnamon, or a whole cinnamon stick
- 2 tsp of Raw Honey or Maple Syrup
- Pinch of Salt
- 1 Tbsp Raisins
- 1 Tsp Vanilla Extract
- ½ Cup + 2 Tbsp Rolled Oats

Optional: ¼ tsp Cardamom, and a pinch of black pepper

Directions

- Combine all ingredients in a sauce pan.

- Turn the stove to medium high and let it cook for about 5 minutes, or until it starts bubbling up.

- Once boiling, remove from heat and cover for 5 minutes.

- Remove the cinnamon stick if you used one, and enjoy hot or cold.

- My daughter loves oats for breakfast, although I leave out the spices for her since she gravitates towards simpler flavors.

Note: If you use a nut milk instead of a rice milk, the oatmeal will be a bit thicker; make sure you do not overcook it as it will burn easily. You can also heat the milk alone with the spices and then once boiling, add the oatmeal, cover, and simmer on low heat for 5 minutes.

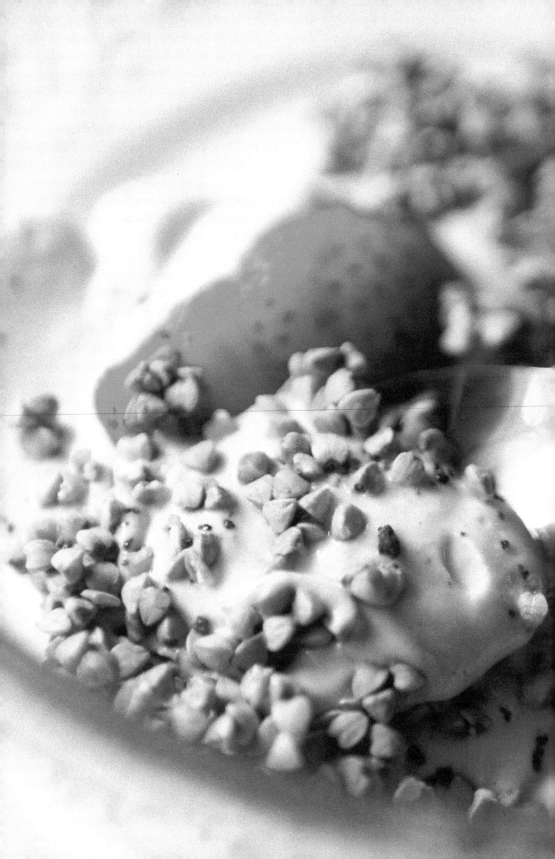

Yogurt

Ingredients

Makes: 2-3 Cups
Portion: Varied

- 2 cups Raw Cashews
- 12 oz Water
- 2 Capsules Probiotics

Other:

- Mason Jar
- Cheesecloth (buy online at Amazon, or at your supermarket)

Directions

- This recipe is a two-step process. The first process consists of letting the yogurt ferment. The second process is to flavor the yogurt.

- We'll start by blending in a high speed blender or Nutribullet the cashews, water and probiotic capsules. You can buy the capsules at a health food store or Whole Foods. It can be one bacteria strain like acidophilus, or you can buy a probiotic that has different strains of bacteria. Choose probiotics that require refrigeration to assure that they are alive and maintained in that condition. To add the capsules to the mix, simple open them with your fingers and deposit the powder into the blender.

- After this is done, pour the yogurt mixture into a mason jar and cover with cheesecloth. Use enough cheesecloth to cover visible openings, though it will still be breathable. I like using a mason jar lid ring to secure the cheese cloth; if not, a rubber band will do.

- Leave the jar in a dark place at room temperature somewhere in your kitchen where it won't get steam from the stove, yet not a completely cold place, or the bacteria won't grow. Leave out for 12 to 24 hours. The longer you leave the jar out, the more time you give the bacteria to grow.
-
- After 12-24 hours, check the yogurt and you will see that it has curdled. If you taste it, it will have that sour yogurt taste, and the yogurt will have a more pure white color than the ivory color of the cashews. If the yogurt has by any chance turned pink, throw it away, a pink color means it has been contaminated.

- Now to flavor the yogurt, pour the mixture back into the blender and add the flavoring agents. Blend and adjust as needed.

- That's how you make plant-based yogurt. You can also substitute coconut meat for cashews!

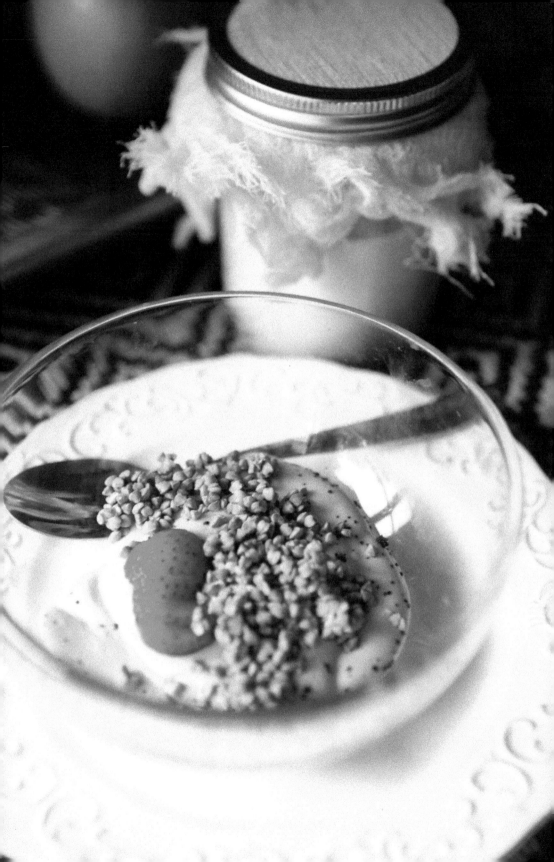

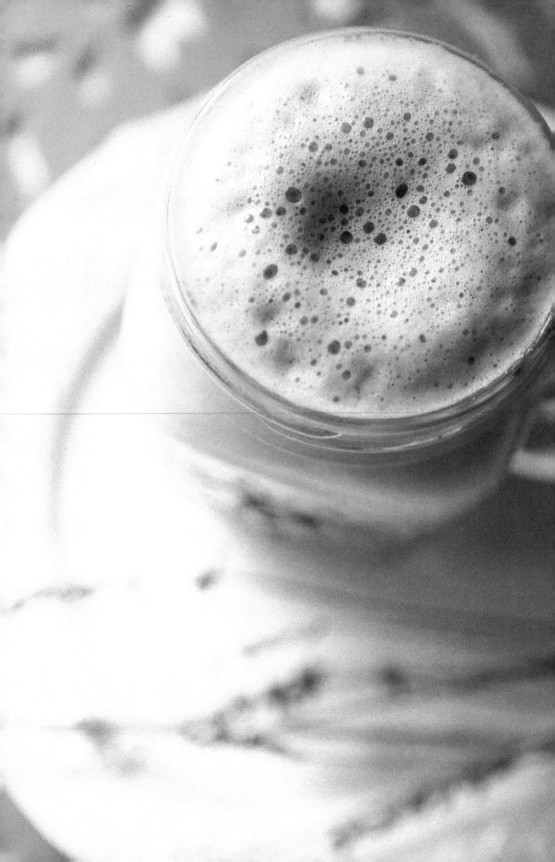

Protein Mochaccino

Ingredients

Makes: 2
Portion: one to one and a half cups

For Tea

- 3 Cardamom Pods
- 1 Cinnamon Stick
- 2" piece of Ginger Root, sliced in half
- 2 Cups Water
- 1 Chicory Tea Bag (optional)

For Mochaccino

- 1 Tbsp Chocolate Protein Powder (I like using Vega brand Chocolate and Greens Protein Powder)
- 1 Tbsp Raw Cashews (optional)

Directions

- In a stove-top tea pot, brew the water with the cardamom, cinnamon, ginger, and chicory tea bag. The chicory tea bag can either be brewed with these ingredients, or its contents can be poured into the blender. Chicory gives the drink a smoky, almost coffee-like flavor. If you don't have a stove-top tea pot, use a small sauce pan.

- Once the tea is brewed, pour all ingredients into a blender, including the chocolate protein powder. Feel free to add cashews if you want a more creamy drink.

- Blend, and pour immediately into your cup for extra foaminess.

- This is my favorite way of drinking my protein drink in the mornings. It's an alternative to a smoothie, that sometimes when taken on an empty stomach can be shocking to our bodies due to the cold temperature.

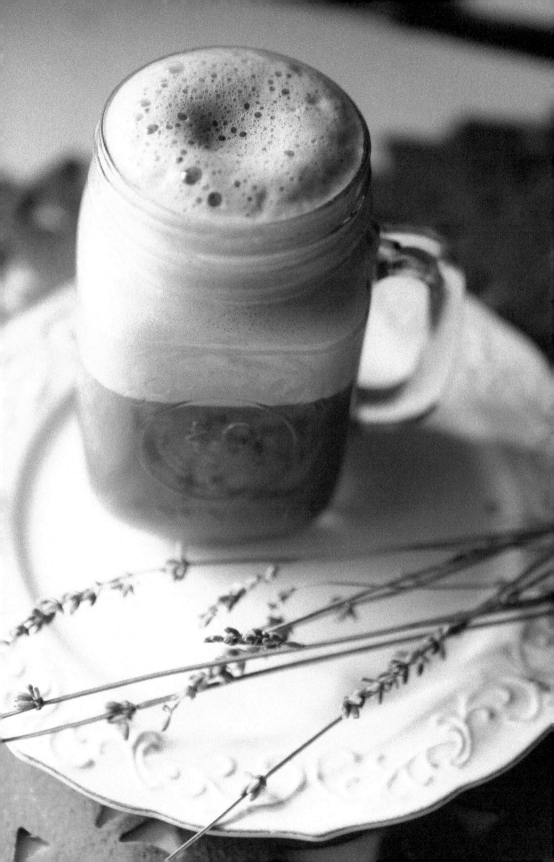

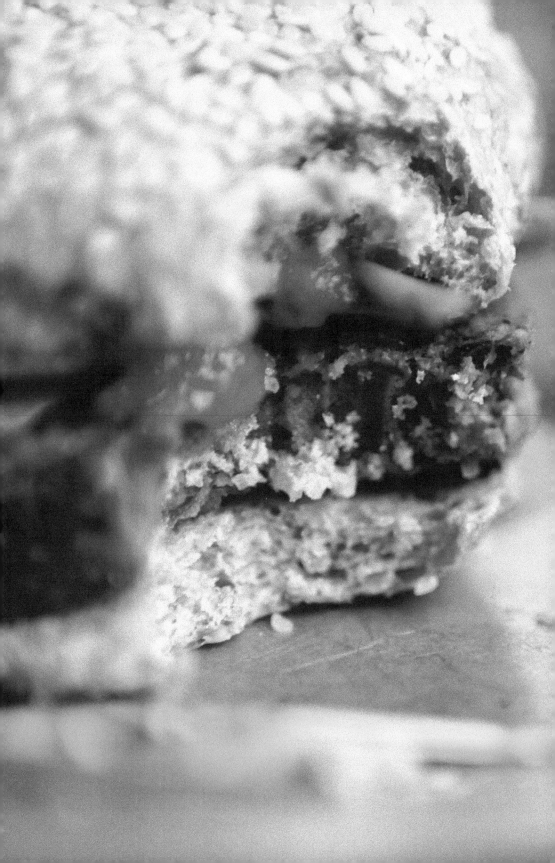

Beet Burger

Ingredients

Makes: 7
Portion: about half a cup

- 2-3 Cloves Garlic, Minced
- 1/2 Onion, Chopped
- 1 Small Red Pepper, Chopped
- 1 Tbsp Mustard (Powder or Sauce)
- 1 Tsp Sea Salt
- 1 Tsp Cumin
- 1 Tsp Paprika
- 2 Tsp Chipotle Pepper Powder
- 1 Tbsp Coconut Aminos
- 1 Cup Shredded Beets
- 1 Can Black Beans
- 1 Cup of Cooked Brown Rice
- 2 Tbsp Sunflower or Nut Butter
- 1 Cup Brown Rice Flour or Oat Flour

Directions

- Heat the skillet to medium heat. Add about one tablespoon of oil; coconut oil or olive oil are fine for this.

- Add the onions and the salt and stir with a wooden spoon a couple of times. We want the onions to get a bit of color, so let them rest without stirring for about a minute or so.

- Then, add the small chopped red pepper, cook for a bit, and add the minced garlic. Sine the pan is warmer than when you added the onions, these last veggies will cook a bit faster, so be vigilant.

- Add the remaining seasonings and stir a couple of times. Once you see the ingredients drying and sticking to the bottom of the pan, lower the heat and add a Tbsp of Coconut Aminos; alternatively you can add Tamari. This process is called deglazing. Use your wooden spoon to gather all the extra flavor that sticks to the bottom of the pan.

- Set aside contents of the skillet.

- In the food processor, shred a cup of beets, then add one cup or one can of black beans and the brown rice. Blend, but keep some of the grainy texture. In other words to do not over-process since the beet has a lot of moisture and will end up liquefying the rest of the ingredients.

- Once processed, transfer to a bowl and add the cooked veggies and the flour to dry up the batter.

- Form the patties to the size and shape desired. Lastly, fry them with a pan and a little oil, or bake for 10 minutes at 350° F, rotating every 5 minutes.

Note: When a recipe calls for a food processor, do not substitute a blender. These two machines are completely different. The food processor is meant to chop, the blender to liquefy. The use of the wrong machine can tremendously affect the end result when making beet burger patties.

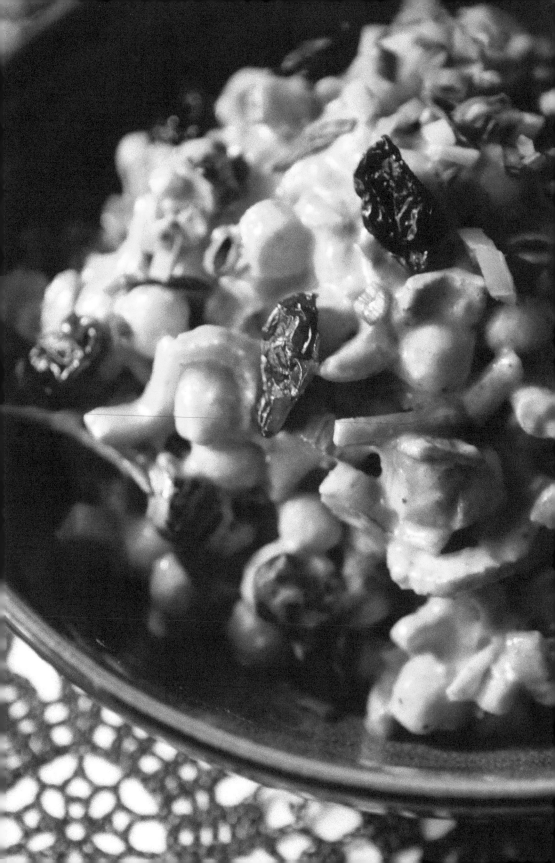

Chickpea Curry Salad

Ingredients

Makes: 4.5 cups
Portion: one cup

For Dressing

- 1 Cup Cashews
- ¼ C Mango Chutney
- ¼ C Rice Vinegar
- 3 Tbsp Curry Powder
- Pinch of Salt
- 6 oz. Water

For Salad

- 1½ C Celery, Chopped Small
- ½ C Green Onions
- 1 Can Chickpeas or 1½ C Cooked Garbanzos
- 1/3 C Cherries or Cranberries
- 1 Tsp of Salt

Directions

- In a blender or Nutribullet, mix all ingredients till smooth and creamy. Be careful not to overheat the cream; if necessary, stop every minute, give it a swirl with a spoon in the blender, and blend again.

- This recipe was given to me by one of my clients, who was given it by her mom, however, we made it plant-based friendly. One of the tricks to assure a delicious curry cream is the brand of curry brand you use. Curry is simply a mix of different spices, so figure out which ones you like best. I prefer a curry with fenugreek and lemon peel in it.

- On the side, chop the veggies small mix with the garbanzos and add the salt. This will make all the vegetables' pores open up so they can absorb the dressing.

- Lastly, pour on the dressing, add the cranberries or cherries, and serve as a side, a salad, or a main dish with a side of grain.

- I always have some dressing left over. I keep it in my fridge for other dishes or to season my butternut squash soup, which is coming up next!

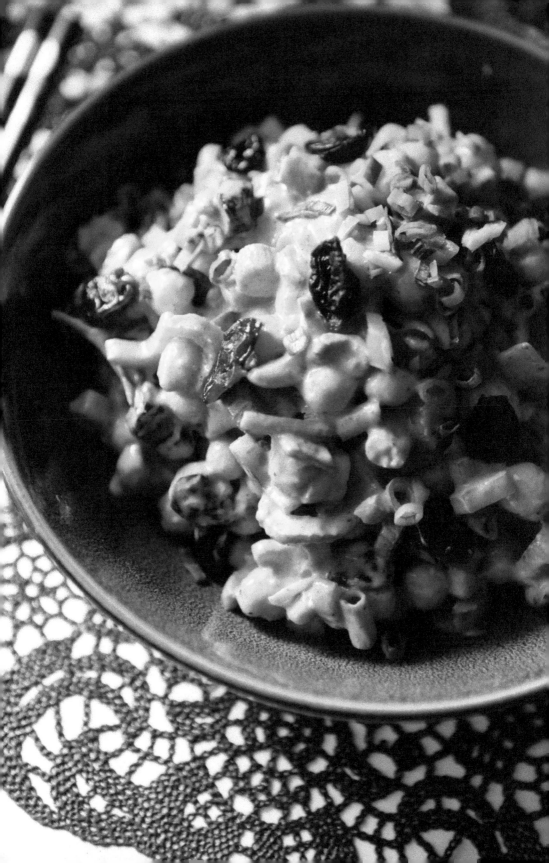

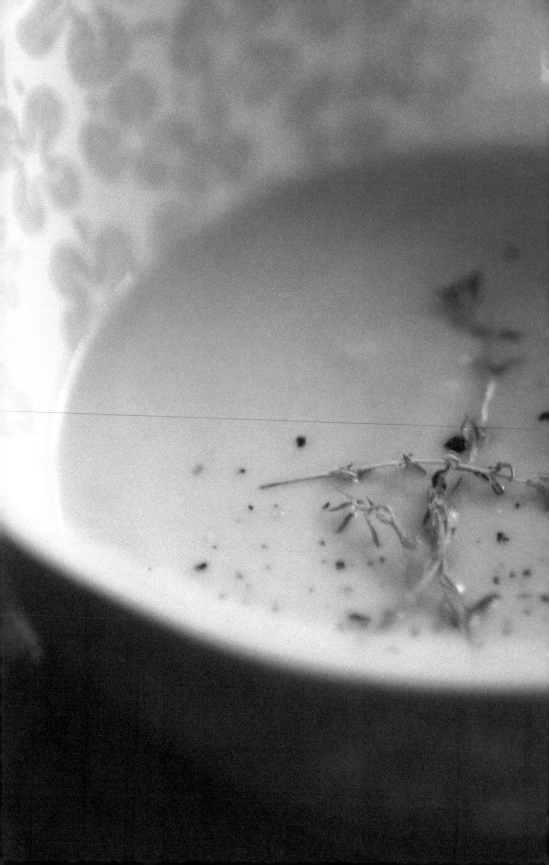

Butternut Squash Soup

Ingredients

Makes: 4-5 Cups
Portion: Varied

- 2 lbs Butternut Squash (This is what a butternut squash in Miami usually weighs; if it is a bit bigger or smaller, it's okay. This is equal to 3 Cups of roasted butternut squash)
- Salt and Pepper to taste
- Coconut Oil or Olive Oil
- 1 Cup Cashews
- 3 C Water
- ½ tsp Salt
- 1 Tsp Lemon Juice

Directions

- A super simple recipe, but it's so delicious and warming. Simply chop the butternut squash into cubes. No need to peel the skin off, just rinse.

- Marinate in a bowl with about one tablespoon of oil, sea salt and pepper.

- Roast in the oven at 400 degrees F for 35–40 minutes, or until the squash is soft to the fork.

- Once roasted, throw in all ingredients into a blender except for the lemon juice, as you don't want to "cook" it in the blender.

- Once creamy, add the lemon juice, taste, and adjust the salt.

- I serve this with a bit of curry cream and crunchy raw buckwheat groats.

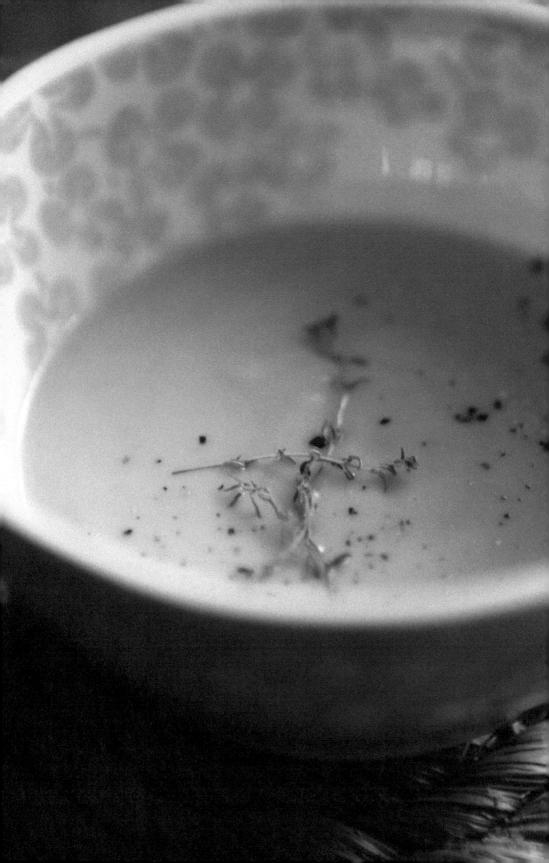

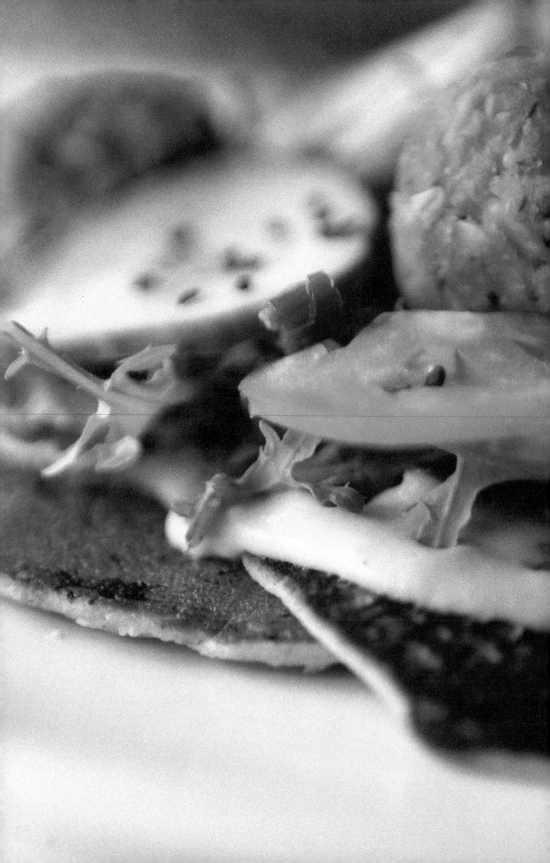

Walnut Balls

Ingredients

Makes: 10
Portion: about one quarter cup

- 1½ Tbsp Olive Oil
- Pink Salt
- 1 Small Yellow Onion – about 1/2 C minced or chopped small
- 1 Red Bell Pepper, diced or chopped small
- 3-4 Garlic Cloves, minced
- 3 Tbsp Dried Basil
- 1-2 Tsps Paprika
- 1 Tsp Red Pepper Flakes (if you like it spicy, if not, omit)
- 1-3 Tbsps Balsamic Vinegar
- 1/2 Cup Walnuts
- 1 Can Chickpeas, or 1-2 Cups of cooked Chickpeas
- 1/4 C Nutritional Yeast

Directions

- Heat a skillet to medium to high heat, add the oil and let it warm up.

- Add the onions and 2–3 pinches of salt. Mix with a wooden spoon, but let the onions rest in the warm pan so that they caramelize a bit. The more mixing you do with the spoon, the more it will create steam, which won't give you the sweet flavor and crunchy texture we want. After they have oozed a bit of their essence into the pan, add the red pepper and the garlic.

- Mix for a bit, let it rest for a bit. Since the pan is warmer they will cook faster and dry out faster too. Have your spices ready to add.

- Add spices, and turn with the spoon a couple of times. If you taste it now, it may taste over seasoned, but that's okay, once we add the chickpeas and nutritional yeast the flavors will even up.

- After a couple stirs, add the walnuts. Cook for about one or two minutes. We want the walnuts to soak up some of the flavor and at the same time ooze some of their oil into the other ingredients.

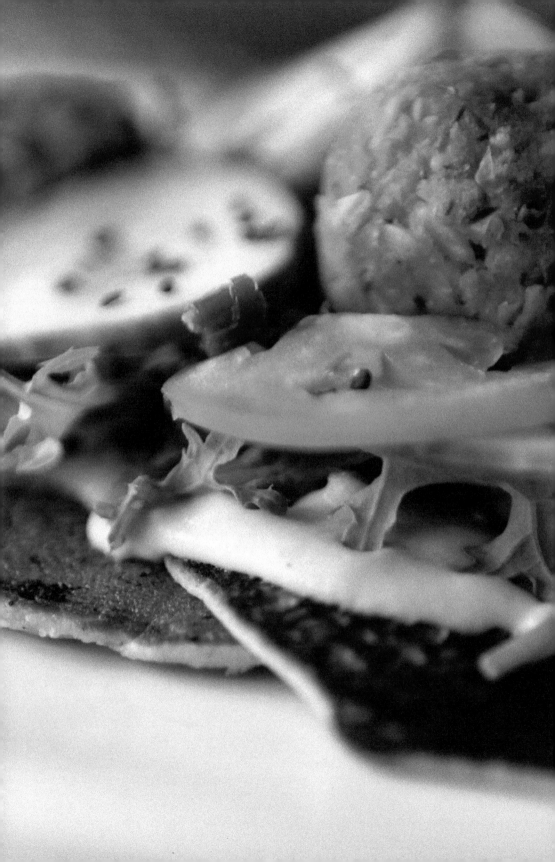

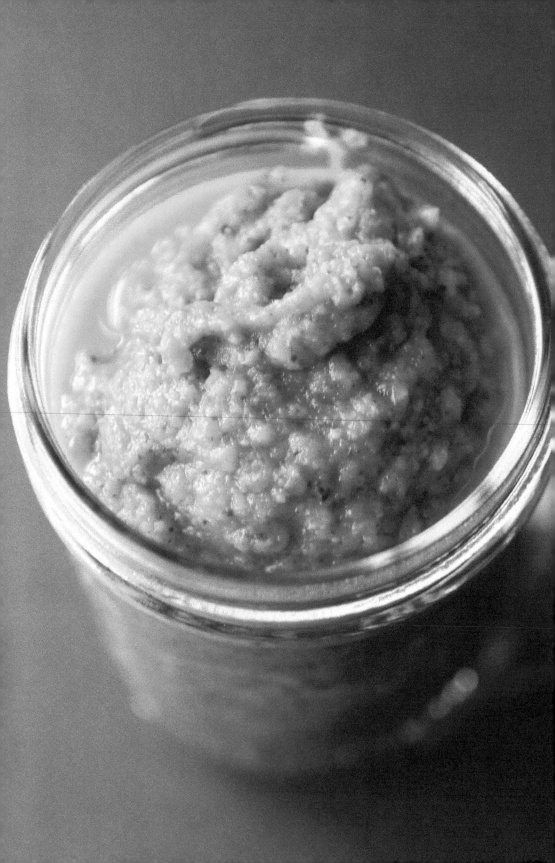

Mushroom Bolognese

Ingredients

Makes: 4 Cups
Portion: Varied

- 1 Tbsp Olive Oil
- 3–4 Pinches Pink Salt to taste
- ½ C Yellow Onion, diced small
- 3–4 Garlic Cloves, minced (chopped very small)
- 3–4 Slim Carrots, coarsely chopped
- 3½ Mushrooms (Shiitake or Crimini preferably)
- 1 Jar Crushed Tomatoes (Jovial Brand)
- ½ C Sundried Tomatoes
- 2–3 Tbsp Dried Basil or 1 clamshell package of Fresh Basil (only the leaves)
- 1½ Tbsp Coconut Sugar

Directions

- In a medium sauce pan, over medium heat, pour in the oil and salt.

- Once hot, add the chopped onion and minced garlic.

- Let it sit in the pan until translucent, then add the dried basil and mix. Note: If using fresh basil, add it at the end with the tomato sauce.

- Add coarsely chopped peeled carrots, sliced mushrooms, and sun-dried tomatoes. Cover and cook for about 5 minutes, stirring occasionally.

- Then add the crushed tomato sauce and coconut sugar. Mix with a spoon to combine all ingredients. Bring it to a boil, then lower the heat to low, cover, and simmer for 15 minutes.

- Check the carrots with a fork; if they are soft, transfer all ingredients to a food processor, if not, simmer for another 5 minutes.

- Once in the food processor, pulse on high a couple times until it has a Bolognese type of texture. Check if there is enough salt. If it still doesn't have a punch of flavor, you can optionally add one more teaspoon of coconut sugar.

Note: To keep your herbs fresh, keep them in an air-tight container covered with a moist paper towel. Store it in the fridge in this way and you can prolong the life of your herbs up to 10 days.

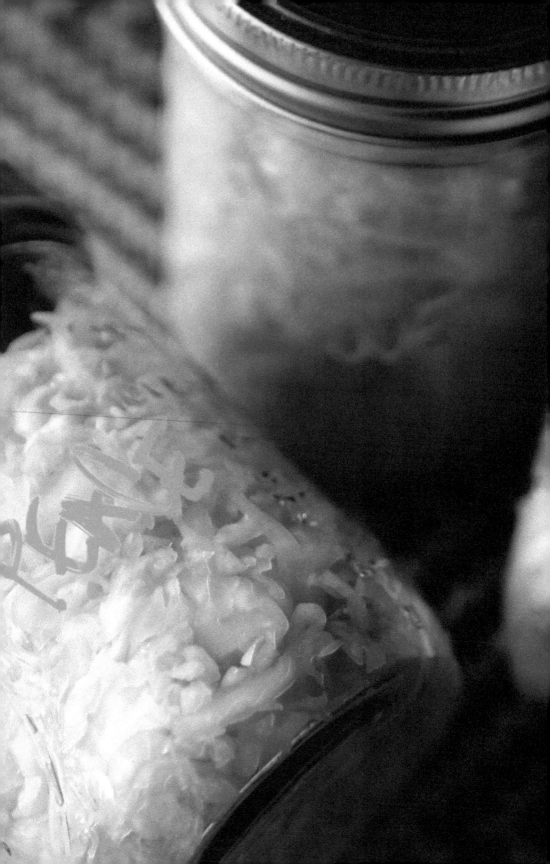

Sauerkraut

Ingredients

Makes: 3 Pints
Portion: 1-2 tablespoons

- 1 Cabbage
- 4 Tsp Mineral Salt

Other:

- Mason Jar

Directions

- Wash your hands and clean the surface you are about to use.

- There are many variants to this recipe, but the basic version uses cabbage. You can add carrots, fennel bulbs, beets, cauliflower, spices, pink peppercorns, or even citrus juices and orange peel. The bottom line is that we are fermenting veggies.

- I find one head of cabbage produces about eight cups of shredded cabbage. For each two cups, I add one teaspoon of mineral salt. The salt is going to wilt the cabbage and make the vegetable ooze its own juice, which we are going to use as a vehicle for fermentation. Cabbage is the go-to vegetable when fermenting, because it already contains numerous wild probiotic strains on its own, so by fermenting it we are creating a place for the bacteria to multiply.

- As you shred the cabbage, every two cups add a teaspoon of salt and massage it with your hands. This makes the process easier, rather than trying to wilt all eight cups of cabbage at the same time.

- Once wilted, put the cabbage in the mason jar, leaving about 1-2" space at the top, so the bacteria have space to breathe. Press the cabbage down with your hands and make sure all the vegetable is submerged under the liquid produced by the vegetable. If it is not enough, add a little water.

- Close the jar tight and label it with the date [and message]. Leave the jar out at room temperature for three days.

- After three days, check the sauerkraut; you'll hear the lid pop, which is a good sign that the bacteria are alive. That's it! Now you can transfer the fermented veggie jar to the fridge and enjoy its wonderful medicinal properties as often as you want.

- You can even swirl the juice of the fermented veggies around in your mouth to restock the good bacteria and protect from the bad.

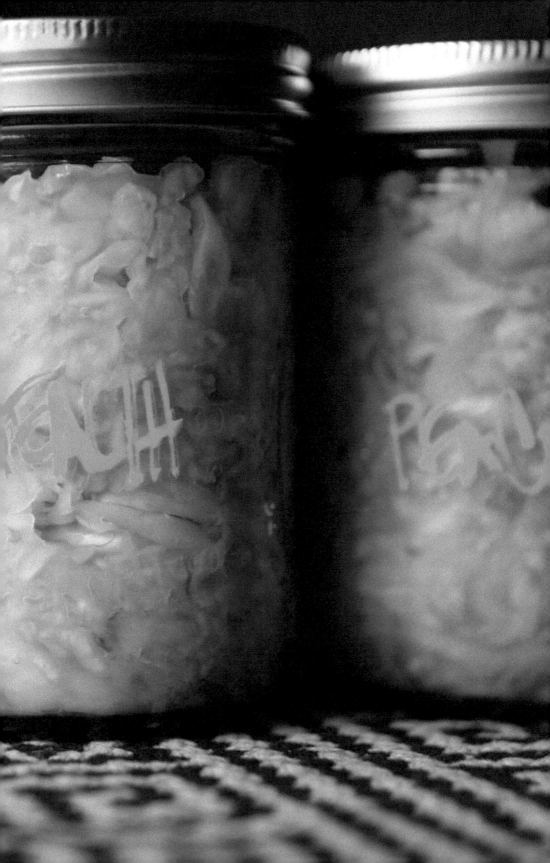

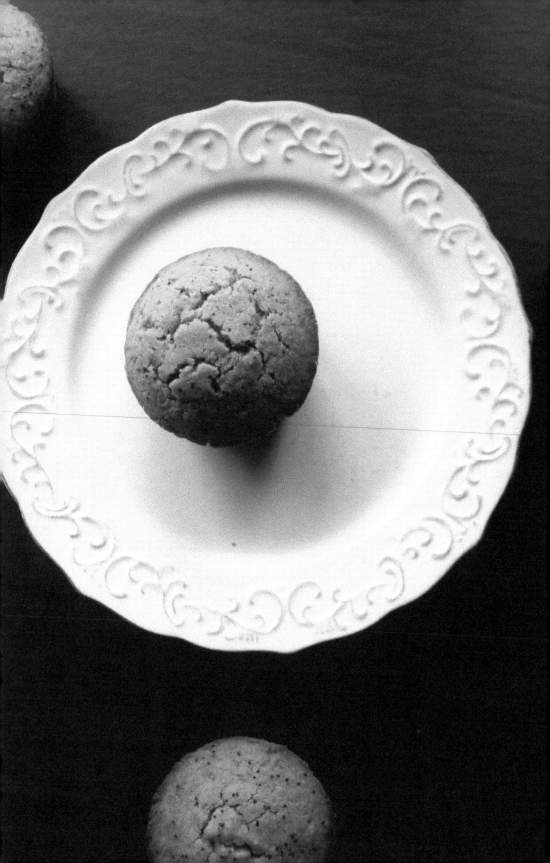

Lemon Poppy Corn Muffin

Ingredients

Makes: 6
Portion: one muffin

- 1 Tbsp Flax Meal whisked with 3 Tbsp Water
- ¼ C Nut Milk or any other Non-Dairy Milk, or your own Cashew Milk!
- 2 Tbsp Lemon Juice
- ¾ C Corn Flour
- ½ C Garbanzo Flour
- ½ Tsp Sea Salt
- ½ Tsp Baking Powder
- ½ Tsp Baking Soda
- Zest of 2 Lemons (The zest is just the yellow skin of the lemons)
- 1 Tbsp Poppy Seeds
- 1 Tbsp Sugar Cane
- 1/8 C Coconut Oil
- ¼ Apple Sauce (Get it out of the fridge in advance so it will not be cold)
- 1/3 C Maple Syrup

Directions

- Preheat oven to 350° F

- Baking is my favorite form of cooking. It's super tricky, however; one extra ounce of flour can throw the entire recipe off. I prefer my baking recipes to be in grams, but since you are doing this at home, I'm giving you the U.S. measurements, but just make sure to be precise with them.

- Also, be sure to follow each step of the recipe in order.

- Make a "flax egg" by whisking the water and the flax meal together in a bowl just big enough to hold the flax egg, and set aside.

- In another small bowl, combine the milk and the lemon juice. Any time you add a vinegar or a citrus to a nut milk it curdles the milk, so this is what we are doing here. Set it aside.

- In another medium bowl, mix all dry ingredients, and add the lemon zest.

- In a medium bowl, add the liquid coconut oil, room temperature apple sauce (since if the apple sauce is cold it will freeze the oil), and maple syrup. Then add the flax egg and whisk a few times.

- Then add the milk, and finally add the dry ingredients to the liquid ingredients bowl.

- With an electric mixer, mix the batter for 3 to 4 minutes at high speed.

- Then divide the batter into six medium size muffin molds. Grease the muffin pan and pour in the batter.

- Bake for 20 minutes.

- Let the muffins cool before removing them from the molds.

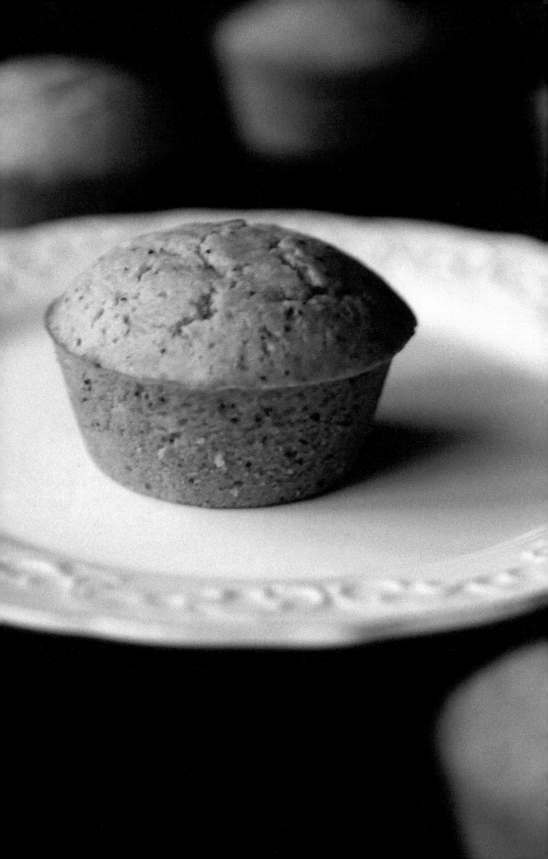

Black Bean Brownies

Ingredients

Makes: 8

- ½ C Coconut Oil
- 1 C Maple Syrup
- 2/3 C Cacao Powder
- ¼ C Apple Sauce
- 2 Individual Packs Instant Coffee, or 1½ Tsp Instant Coffee
- 2 oz very HOT Water
- ¼ Tsp Baking Powder
- 1 Tsp Pink Salt
- 3 Cups Cooked Black Beans (mushy)
- 3 Tbsp Turbinado Sugar
- 1½ C Rolled Oats

Optional: 1/3 Cup Chocolate Chips

Directions

- If you have a powerful blender, use it. If not, use a food processor.

- It's important to first blend the oil, maple syrup, and cacao powder.

- Then, dissolve the instant coffee in hot water and add it to the blender with the salt and baking powder. Then add the black beans; blend until smooth.

- Lastly, add the turbinado sugar and the oats to the blender. Pulse or blend; you should still be able to see traces of the oats in the batter, it doesn't have to be completely blended.

- Transfer to a greased 8x8 brownie pan, add chocolate chips, and mix with a spoon.

- Bake for 25 minutes at 350° F. Turn the pan after 25 minutes and bake for five minutes more.

- The brownies at this point will be slightly wet in the middle, but they'll dry out as it cools down.

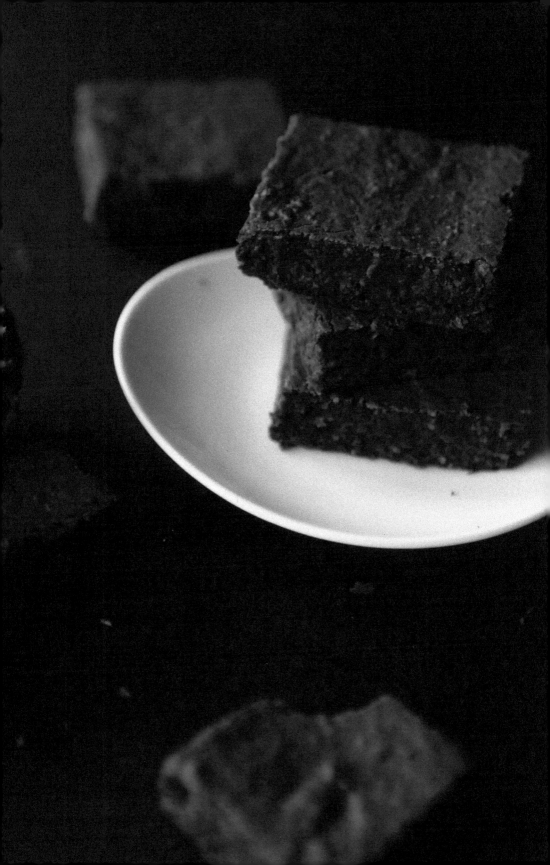

Acknowledgments

Every time I thank the Earth I'm thanking you, mother. Every time I thank the Universe, I'm thanking you, Dad. Through your union and your love you offered me a portal to bring me here to the world. We've had our issues, discussions, and complete disagreements on many things, but in all of the challenges that you presented me, love always reigned. Those moments of critical thinking made me stronger, which pushed me to search for a better understanding and perhaps a change of perspective. Because of you, I am who I am. Mother, I thank you for your patience and your unconditional love. Dad, I've always admired your devotion to service. Thank you for instilling these values in me that have led me to write about this path.

Esperanza, thank you for showing me the true spelling of hope : wisdom.

Pollo and J, thank you for your unbreakable strength.

Mango, thank you for sprouting a book out of me.

Muñeka, my companion.

Violetta Sky, for life.

Alex, teacher.

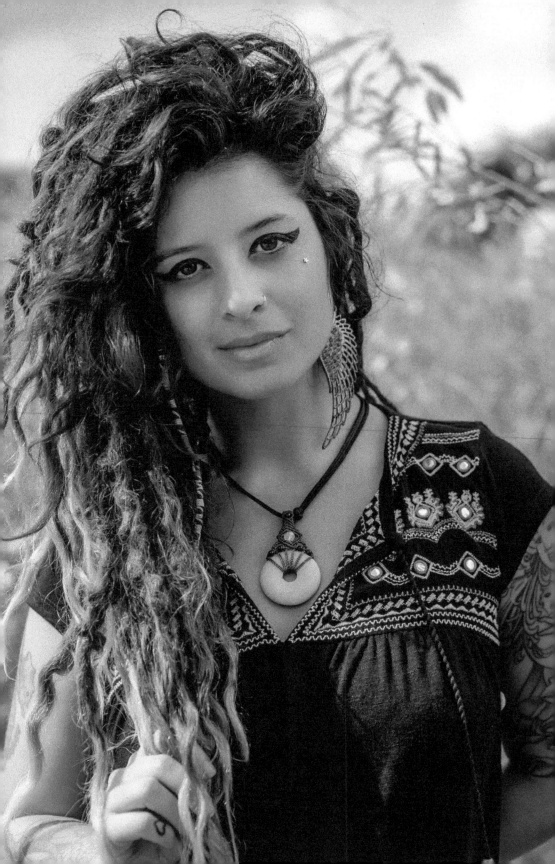

Author Bio

Pamela Wasabi is a lead authority in the plant-based and wellness communities of Miami. She is most recognized for hosting and preparing farm-to-table vegan dinners, supporting local agriculture, and leading workshops and lectures on our relationship with food, nourishment, and sacred femininity. Her background stretches from holistic nutrition and the psychology of eating to plant-based cuisine. It is her mission to awaken the collective consciousness into living in harmony with Nature.

Wasabi has been cooking in a plant-based way since 2013. Her culinary quest began when she encountered a medical diagnosis that impeded her from having a natural birth and sentenced her to be on prescription pills for the rest of her life. She escaped this medical trap by studying holistic nutrition, learning how to cook, and expanding her practice as a health educator by pursuing the studies at the Institute for the Psychology of Eating. Halfway through her nine-month cycle, she balanced her hormones and thyroid condition by simply changing the way she approached food, the ingredients selected, and the nourishment she offered herself by cooking her own meals. After giving birth to her daughter, what started as a hobby became her full-time career. She currently manages her two-stream company, a wholesale line of gluten free and baked goods, and a meal prep service titled Nourished Cuisine. Wasabi is also in practice as a health/eating counselor.

CPSIA information can be obtained
at www.ICGtesting.com
Printed in the USA
BVHW021125201219
567074BV00002B/1/P